GW00372455

DEPARTMENT OF TRANSPORT

Transport Statistics Report

ROAD ACCIDENT STATISTICS
ENGLISH REGIONS 1995

Published August 1996

London: HMSO

Prepared for publication by STD5 branch
Strategy and Analysis Unit
Department of Transport

Jonathan Martin
Paul O'Connor
Linden Francis

GOVERNMENT STATISTICAL SERVICE

A service of statistical information and advice is provided to the government by specialist staff employed in the statistics divisions of individual Departments. Statistics are made generally available through their publications and further information and advice on them can be obtained from the Departments concerned.

Enquiries about the contents of this publication should be made to:

Department of Transport
SAU, STD5 Division
1st Floor
Great Minster House
76 Marsham Street
London SW1P 4DR

Telephone 0171 271 3829
Telephone 0171 276 8785 (Prior to 16th September 1996)

Data Service

Copies of the main tables in this publication can be supplied on a computer diskette by the Department of Transport (at a cost of £40). Further tabulations of road accident statistics are also available from the Department, subject to confidentiality rules. The charges vary with the complexity of the analysis (minimum £40 per data run) and the availability of these services depends upon the resources within the Department. Enquiries should be addressed in writing to Mr P S O'Connor at the above address

Acknowledgements
The Department of Transport would like to acknowledge the assistance provided by the Police Accident Investigation Unit at Catford.

Contents

Symbols and Conventions

Rounding of Figures:

In tables where figures have been rounded there may be an apparent slight discrepancy between the sum of the constituent items and the independently rounded total.

Symbols:

.. = not available

Conversion Factor:

1 kilometre = 0.6214 mile

Preface

This edition of Road Accident Statistics English Regions (RASER) gives statistics of road accidents on a local basis for England in the years up to 1995. RASER concentrates on accidents as being incidents which may reflect a need for local action and is intended to be of most benefit to traffic engineers, planners and administrators in local government and the Government Offices for the Regions. For this reason, most of the data in the book are compiled according to the county groupings covered by these offices.

RASER includes only background national statistics, so it should be regarded as a supplement to "Road Accidents Great Britain 1995 - The Casualty Report" (RAGB), which is the main publication on road accident statistics in Great Britain. RAGB 1995 is available from HMSO bookshops, price £13.00.

The current system of collecting road accident statistics was set up in 1968, and is for the benefit and use of local authorities, the police and central government. Each year, about 230,000 STATS19 road accident report forms (an example of which can be found on pages 56 to 58) are completed by police officers of the 51 police forces in Great Britain. These forms record data about accidents on the public highway which involved personal injury or death. These data are transferred onto magnetic tape or computer diskette and are sent to DOT where they are incorporated into an annual data file.

The principal purpose in collecting and publishing statistics of road accidents is to provide background information for both central government and local authorities about the roads, road users, locations, times of day, weather conditions, etc involved in road accidents, and against which various remedial measures can be considered. Road accident statistics are used to provide both a local and a national perspective for particular road safety problems or particular suggested remedies. A continuous flow of information - such as the time series tables in this book - means that trends of accidents and casualties can be examined and used to change the direction of policies when necessary.

The report also includes data from Northern Ireland. These data, where available, are included with each table along with data for Scotland and Wales. *More detailed statistics for Scotland and Wales are available from the Scottish and Welsh Offices - please refer to the inside rear cover for more details.*

Several of the tables contain averages of 1981-85 data. These represent the base figures which the Secretary of State for Transport used to set the target of reducing the number of road casualties by one third by the year 2000. It should also be noted that main Tables 1 and 6 which give casualty totals by severity for the years covering 1981 to 1985 have been extended to show revised estimates for London for this period. At the beginning of September 1984 the Metropolitan police implemented improved procedures for allocating the level of severity to accidents and casualties. The change is thought to have had no effect on overall casualty numbers, but in the period between 1981 and the date of the change it is estimated that there were 4,725 casualties whose injuries were originally judged to be slight but would have been judged serious under the later procedures. However, this is an overall estimate and it is not possible to present similar revised estimates of accidents by road type and other detailed characteristics.

DOT is generally prepared to sell tabulations of road accident data. The cost of data varies with the complexity of each request, but averages about £40 per data run. Further information can be obtained from: - *Mr Paul O'Connor, Department of Transport, 1st Floor, Great Minster House, 76 Marsham Street, London, SW1P 4DR, Telephone 0171-271-3829.*

1. Commentary on tables and charts

Jonathan Martin, Strategy and Analysis Unit, Department of Transport

Introduction

This section gives a review of the tables and charts included in this report. As noted in the preface, and with the exception of table 15, the data are disaggregated either by county, Government Office (GO) region, or Highways Agency (HA) region. Northern Ireland data have been included within certain tables and those tables where Northern Ireland data are not available, and thus where no United Kingdom total can be given, have been individually annotated.

From April 1994, the DOT regional offices were subsumed within the Government Offices for regions (GORs). This edition of RASER uses the GORs as the basis for its regional breakdowns for the first time. In order to provide consistent time series, wherever data for earlier years are shown in the tables, these are also on the basis of the new GOR definition. Note however that the regional figures given in this edition will not be consistent with those published in earlier editions. A map showing the GORs can be found on page 51.

This publication follows Government Statistical Service advice in showing data for the Merseyside GOR both separately and combined with the neighbouring North West GOR. However the Merseyside GOR is much smaller in terms of area, population and traffic than other Government Office regions, therefore it is often not appropriate to make direct comparisons with these other regions. This article refers to the Merseyside GOR when commenting on rates, proportions and extreme cases, but not when discussing absolute numbers of accidents or casualties.

The Highways Agency is responsible for the construction and management of motorways and trunk roads in England. Until April 1994, the management function was carried out by nine Network Management Divisions, covering the same areas as the Department's old Regional Offices. However during 1994, the Agency reduced the number of Network Management Divisions to four, covering wider areas. To cater for this change, an Annex has been added to this edition of RASER. Each table from the main body of the report which contains statistics for the GORs is repeated in this Annex, showing equivalent figures for the Highways Agency Network Management Division Regions. Tables 2, 4, 5 and 6 from the main report which analyse casualty data by county reproduce the same analysis in the Annex, but only for Highways Agency Regions instead of counties. Unless the table headings state otherwise, these tables show data for all road accidents in these regions, not just those occurring on roads for which the Highways Agency is responsible. A map showing the Highways Agency regions can be found on page 53.

It should also be noted that population figures used in this report are final mid-1994 estimates. Mid-year estimates for 1995 were not available at the time of going to publication.

Casualties

Table 1 gives the regional distribution of casualties and is presented as a time series for the period 1988 to 1995. The average for the years 1981-1985 is also given. There has been little significant change in the aggregate casualty distribution between the regions over this period. In each of the eight years shown, London had the highest number of casualties. Throughout this period, the South East region, had the next highest number of casualties. By 1995 the number of casualties in the South East region, was only slightly less than for London. Excluding Merseyside from the comparison of casualty levels, the lowest number of casualties was in the North East, which had total casualties less than half of any other region.

The table also shows that in 1995 London had the highest overall casualty rate per 100,000 population, followed by Merseyside and the North West region. The lowest rates were found in the North East and South West regions. London, however, had the lowest fatality rate of all the regions - probably because accidents in urban areas tend to be less severe because they occur at lower speeds. The highest fatality rate was in the East Midlands region with the next highest in the South West and Eastern regions.

Chart 1a depicts the number of casualties killed and the number seriously injured in each region in 1995. The chart shows that the East Midlands, North West/Merseyside and the South East regions had the highest number of those killed and London and the South East region the highest number of those seriously injured.

Chart 1b depicts the number of casualties killed or seriously injured (KSI) and slightly injured in each region in 1995 and shows that London had the highest number of casualties in both severity groups and the North East the lowest number.

Chart 2 depicts the number of child casualties per 100,000 child population in each region in 1995 and shows that Scotland had the highest rate of children killed or seriously injured and the South East and South West regions the lowest rate. Merseyside had the highest overall rate of child casualties.

Chart 3 shows the number of adult casualties per 100,000 adult population in each region in 1995 and shows that the East Midlands region had the highest rate of adults killed or seriously injured and Merseyside the lowest rate. The North West and Merseyside regions had the highest overall rate of adult casualties.

Charts 4 and **5** depict the percentage change in overall casualties and those killed or seriously injured for each region between 1994 and 1995 (the charts take account of the change in regional definition as noted in the introduction). **Chart 4** shows that overall casualties have decreased in all but two of the thirteen regions (including Wales and Scotland). The increases being in the North East and South West regions, but of less than half of one per cent. **Chart 5** shows that casualties killed or seriously injured fell in eight English regions, as well as in Wales and Scotland. Both Merseyside and the West Midlands regions recorded decreases of over ten per cent. There was an increase of over five per cent in both the East Midlands and London regions.

4

Local authority casualty comparisons

Tables 2-5 give information on the number of casualties, rate per 100,000 population, and percentage distribution, by age and road user type for each English county, Scotland and Wales.

Table 2 gives the number of casualties by age and road user type for 1995 and **Table 3** gives the same information as an average for the years 1981-1985.

Table 4 gives casualty rates, per 100,000 population, by age and by type of road user for each English county. In England in 1995, 376 children were killed or injured in road accidents per 100,000 children and the county casualty rates varied from 267 in Avon to 493 in Merseyside. The casualty rate for those aged 60 and over varied from 203 in Avon to 351 in North Yorkshire. The overall casualty rate for all ages was lowest in Tyne & Wear and highest in Surrey. The pedestrian casualty rate was highest in most urbanised areas, in particular London and Greater Manchester, and lowest in rural counties such as Oxfordshire, Somerset and Suffolk. The pedal cyclist casualty rate was highest in Cambridgeshire and lowest in Durham and Northumberland. The car occupant casualty rate varied from 245 in Avon to 516 in Surrey.

Table 5 gives the distribution of casualties, by age and by type of road user, for each county. In England in 1995, 14 per cent of road accident casualties were children and 10 per cent were aged 60 and over. The proportion of casualties who were children varied from 10 per cent in Surrey to 19 per cent in Cleveland. The Isle of Wight had the highest proportion of casualties aged 60 or over; 18 per cent compared with 10 per cent in the whole of England.

Table 6 gives the number of casualties killed or seriously injured and total casualties in each English county for 1995 and compares them with the average for the years 1981-1985. The percentage change is also given. In England as a whole, the number killed or seriously has fallen by 38 per cent and overall casualties by 2.5 per cent. The number of casualties killed or seriously injured has fallen in every county except Cheshire, with the largest fall, at 70 per cent, recorded in Berkshire. The large variation in the change in total casualties since the baseline between counties will reflect the effects of any changes to reporting procedures during this period.

Casualties by road type

Charts 6a and **6b** depict the number of casualties killed or seriously injured and slightly injured in each region on built-up and non built-up roads respectively. On built-up roads, the highest number of casualties for both severity groups was in London, with the North East and Wales having the lowest number for both severity groups. On non built-up roads, the highest number of casualties both killed or seriously injured and slightly injured were in the South East region. Scotland and the Eastern region also had high numbers of casualties killed or seriously injured. The lowest number of casualties for both severity groups was in London.

Table 7 gives the total number of casualties in each region disaggregated by severity and by road type. In most regions well over 50 per cent of casualties were in accidents on built-up roads. In London the figure was 96% whereas in the Eastern region, the figure was only 54%. The South East region had the highest proportion of casualties on motorways, with 6%. Of the other regions only the North West and the Eastern region had greater than 5% of their casualties on motorways. The proportion of casualties who were killed or seriously injured was highest on non built-up roads. The highest proportion was in Yorkshire/Humberside and the East Midlands region, where 23% of casualties were killed or seriously injured. The East Midlands also had the highest proportion of KSI to all casualties on built-up roads.

Charts 7 and **8** show, for built-up and non built-up roads respectively, overall casualty numbers on trunk, principal and other roads in each region in 1995. On built-up roads, the highest number of casualties on trunk, principal and other roads was in London. The South East also had a large number of casualties on other roads. The number of trunk road casualties in London was almost five times the size of trunk road casualties in any of the other regions. On non built-up roads the highest number of casualties on trunk roads was in the Eastern region. The highest number of casualties on principal and other roads was in the South East region.

Table 8 gives the casualty rates by severity for motorways and A roads for each region. The casualty rate is derived by dividing the number of casualties on a particular road type by the traffic carried on those roads. The rates are given as an average for the period 1993 to 1995. The highest rate for total casualties on motorways, was in London with the lowest rate being in the South West. The fatality rate on motorways deviated only slightly between the majority of the regions, however the highest was in the North East, where the rate was twice as high as any other region. London and Merseyside had the highest rate for total casualties on all A roads, with the South West having the lowest rate. For England as a whole, the highest total casualties rate was on built-up trunk and principal roads, and the lowest on motorways.

Accidents

Table 9 gives accident rates by severity for motorways and A roads for each region. The accident rate is derived by dividing the number of accidents on particular road types by the traffic carried on that road type. The rates are given as an average for the period 1993 to 1995. In England over the three year period, built-up principal A roads had the highest all severities accident rate at 101 accidents per 100 million vehicle kilometres. Motorways had the lowest rate, at 11 accidents per 100 million vehicle kilometres. For fatal accidents, the respective rates for these two road types were 1.0 accidents and 0.2 accidents.

Chart 9 depicts the number of accidents on motorways and trunk and principal A roads in each region in 1995. The South East and North West regions, had the highest number of accidents on motorways, whilst London had the highest number of accidents on trunk and principal A roads.

Seasonal pattern of accidents

The seasonal pattern of injury accidents is given in **Table 10**. The base has been calculated as the average number of accidents per day in each region. The peak months for accidents can vary from year to year for various reasons, for example, differing weather conditions. In 1995 the general pattern is low accident rates in the early part of the year building to a peak from September to November. Several regions however had smaller peaks in June and July. The pattern within the two metropolitan regions of London and Merseyside fluctuated greatly and did not reflect the general trend across England. The peak month in 1995 for the all severity accident rate was either November or September for all of the regions. For the fatal or serious accident rate, the same was true with the exception of London and Merseyside whose peaks were October and March respectively. The lowest accident rate occurred during April for all regions except Merseyside whose lowest all severity accident rate occurred in June. The lowest fatal and serious accident rate varied a great deal, however with the exception of two regions, it occurred in the first half of the year.

Accidents by road type

Tables 11-13 show the number of junction and non-junction injury accidents occurring on motorways and trunk and principal A roads. On all motorways in England, 17 per cent of accidents occurred at junctions and roundabouts this figure was 59 per cent on all trunk A roads and 69 per cent on all principal A roads.

Regionally accidents at junctions and roundabouts accounted for about 50 per cent of all trunk road accidents. For the North West and West Midlands regions, the corresponding figure was around sixty five per cent and seventy per cent for London. For principal A roads, the proportion of accidents at junctions and roundabouts was higher than for trunk roads. For all regions except the South West, North West and London, the figure was around sixty five per cent. 72 per cent of accidents occurred at junctions/roundabouts in the North west and 78 per cent in London. The South West region had the lowest proportion with 59 per cent.

The proportion of fatal or serious accidents on junctions and at roundabouts was around ten per cent less than the all severities proportion except in London where for both trunk and principal roads, there was little difference between accident severities.

Table 14 gives the total number of injury accidents disaggregated by severity on different types of road in each region and county for 1994 and 1995. The average for the years 1981 to 1985 is also given. The road classifications used are motorways, trunk and principal A roads and all roads.

Table 15 shows injury accidents and casualties by severity, and the vehicles involved, for individual English motorways, including A(M) roads. Eighty four per cent of the vehicles involved were cars or vans while 13 per cent were heavy lorries, broadly in line with their share of motorway traffic. Motorways with the highest numbers of accidents per kilometre in 1995 were the M25 (5.5 accidents) and the M63 (5.1 accidents).

Table 16 gives the percentage of accidents on the various types of road within each region. This table should be considered in conjunction with Table 19 which shows the distribution of motor traffic within each region.

Background data

Table 17 gives regional background information on road lengths, home population, area, and licensed vehicle numbers. **Table 18** gives the 1993-1995 average distribution between regions of motor traffic on major roads, and **Table 19** shows the distribution of motor traffic within each region. All road lengths shown in Tables 15 and 17 are taken from the Transport Statistics Report *"Road Lengths in Great Britain 1995"*.

List of charts and tables

CHARTS

Chart 1a: Fatal and serious casualties: by region: 1995

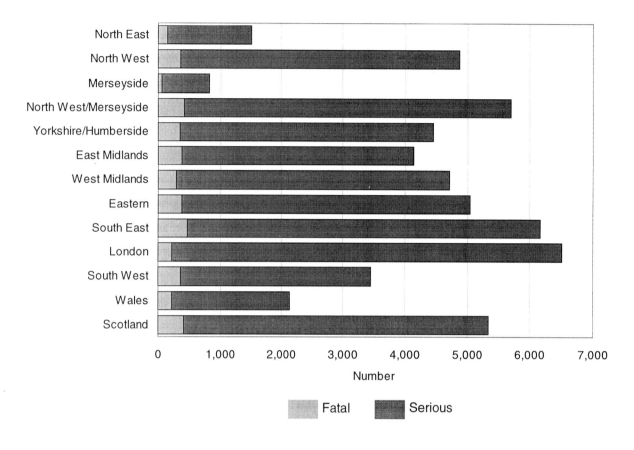

Number

Fatal   Serious

Chart 1b: KSI and slight casualties: by region: 1995

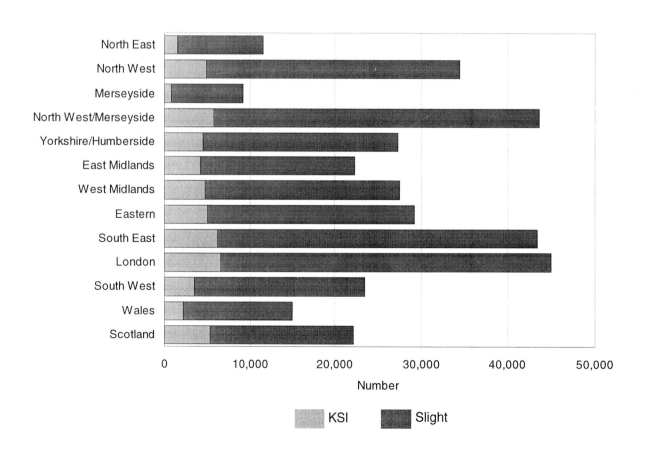

Number

KSI   Slight

Chart 2: Child casualtes per 100,000 child population: by severity and region: 1995

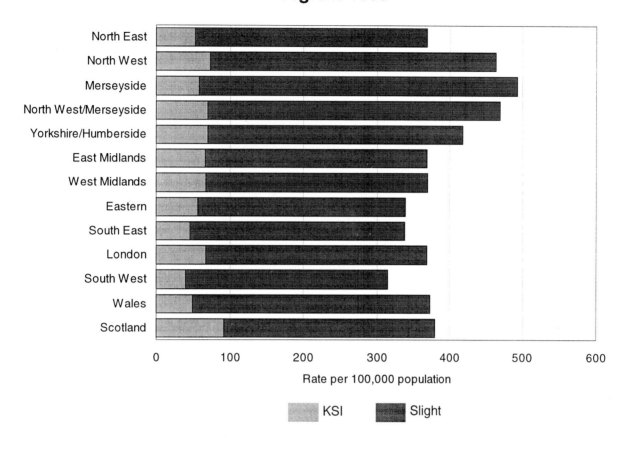

Rate per 100,000 population

KSI   Slight

Chart 3: Adult casualties per 100,000 adult population: by severity and region: 1995

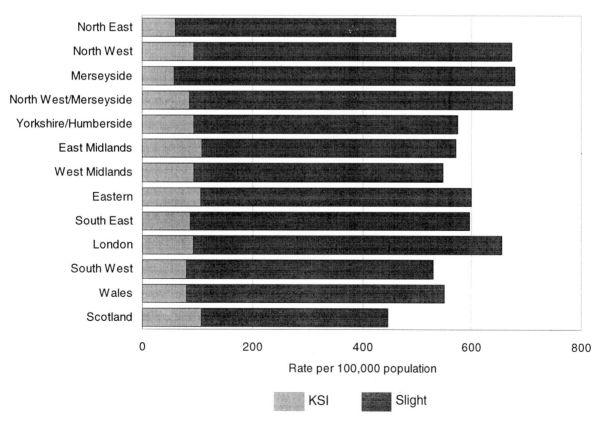

Rate per 100,000 population

KSI   Slight

Chart 4: Percentage change in total casualties: by region: 1994-1995

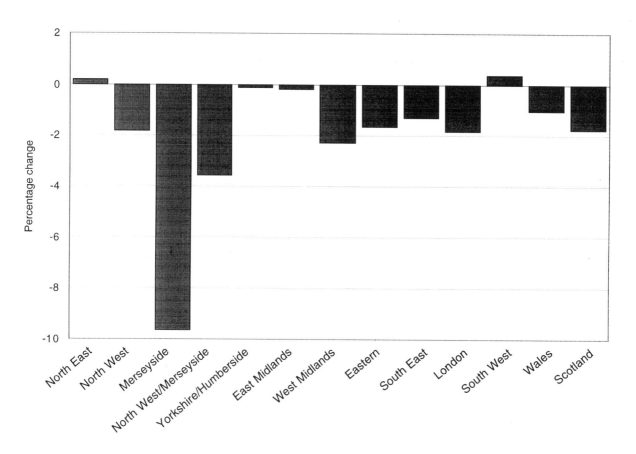

Chart 5: Percentage change in KSI casualties: by region: 1994-1995

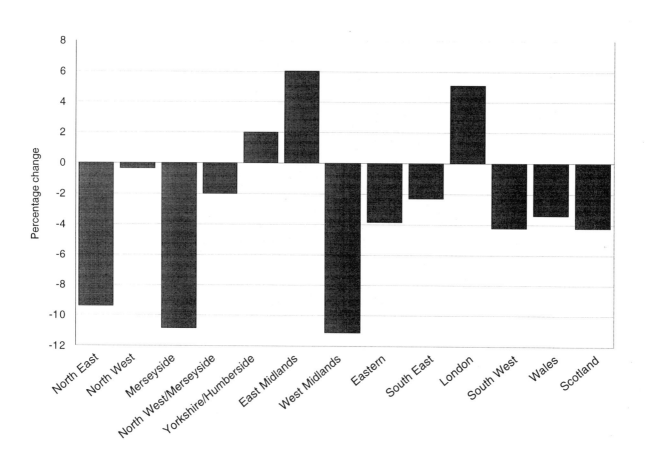

Chart 6a: Casualties on built-up roads: by severity and region: 1995

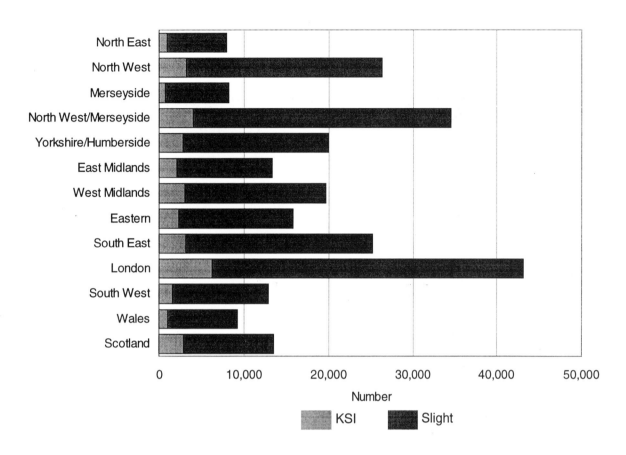

Chart 6b: Casualties on non built-up roads: by severity and region: 1995

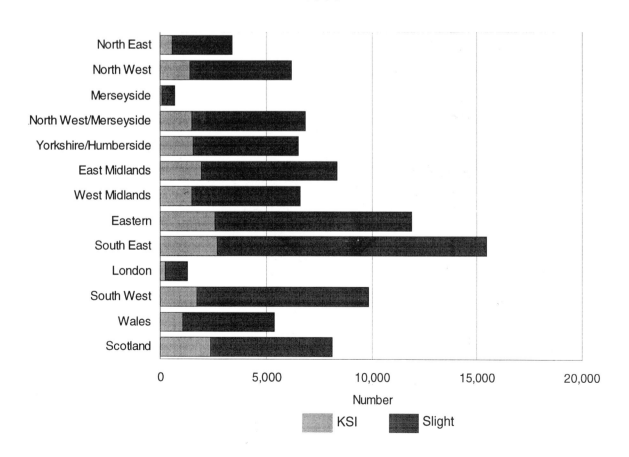

Chart 7: Casualties by road class and region: built-up roads: 1995

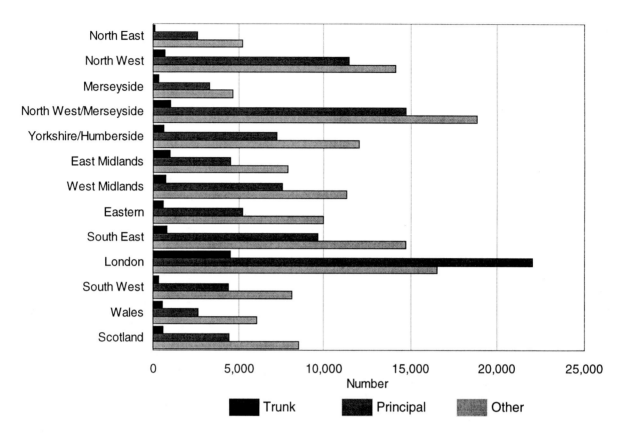

Chart 8: Casualties by road class and region: non built-up roads: 1995

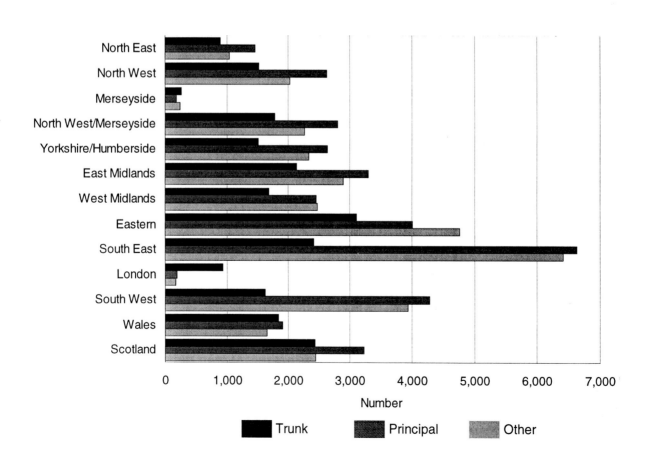

Chart 9: Accidents by road class and region: 1995

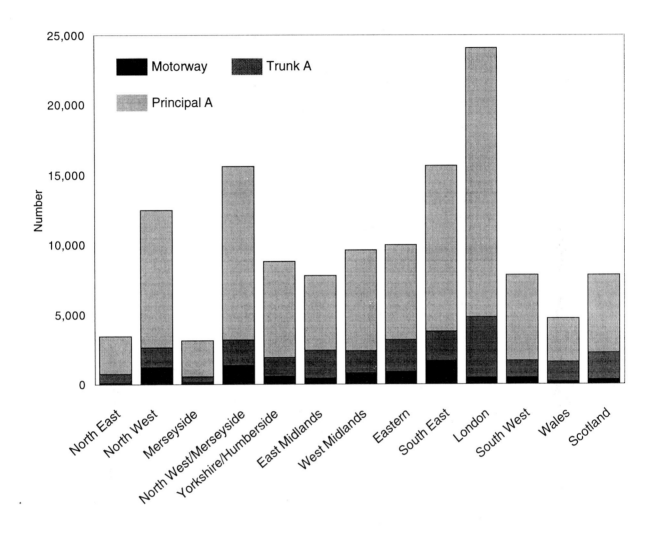

TABLES

1 Casualties: by Government Office Region and severity: 1981-85 average, 1988-1995: rate per 100,000 population, 1995

Number/rate

		1981-85 Average	1988	1989	1990	1991	1992	1993	1994	1995	Rate per 100,000 Population[1]
North East	Fatal	221	213	210	246	212	161	169	132	152	5.8
	KSI	2,637	2,260	2,248	2,271	2,043	1,910	1,690	1,673	1,516	58.1
	Total	11,107	11,208	12,741	13,001	12,241	11,935	11,262	11,491	11,514	441.2
North West	Fatal	486	454	475	494	449	424	369	350	358	6.5
	KSI	5,810	4,830	4,993	5,155	4,452	4,306	4,195	4,892	4,875	89.2
	Total	29,058	30,975	33,142	34,238	31,805	32,837	32,691	35,085	34,447	630.0
Merseyside	Fatal	114	111	97	81	94	77	71	76	60	4.2
	KSI	1,237	1,029	1,055	1,094	1,128	1,070	998	923	823	57.4
	Total	7,225	8,221	8,917	9,511	9,816	10,141	10,437	10,151	9,173	639.5
North West/Merseyside	Fatal	600	565	572	575	543	501	440	426	418	6.1
	KSI	7,047	5,859	6,048	6,249	5,580	5,376	5,193	5,815	5,698	82.6
	Total	36,284	39,196	42,059	43,749	41,621	42,978	43,128	45,236	43,620	632.0
Yorkshire/Humberside	Fatal	501	437	480	428	413	414	387	325	345	6.9
	KSI	6,830	6,131	6,127	5,978	5,202	5,110	4,603	4,357	4,444	88.4
	Total	25,915	26,884	28,560	28,455	26,086	26,599	26,031	27,310	27,279	542.8
East Midlands	Fatal	492	413	514	513	410	393	350	341	378	9.2
	KSI	6,389	5,031	5,342	5,045	4,173	4,145	3,940	3,905	4,140	100.9
	Total	23,079	23,308	25,129	24,852	22,397	22,175	22,207	22,375	22,331	544.3
West Midlands	Fatal	525	442	498	478	386	395	353	382	286	5.4
	KSI	7,854	5,771	6,190	6,136	5,298	4,913	4,514	5,303	4,713	89.0
	Total	27,691	26,753	28,964	30,219	27,425	27,089	26,599	28,114	27,473	518.8
Eastern	Fatal	533	524	556	544	493	425	402	391	374	7.2
	KSI	8,281	7,537	7,318	7,026	5,846	5,648	5,242	5,242	5,040	96.5
	Total	30,288	34,090	35,442	33,973	30,119	29,537	29,510	29,749	29,253	560.0
South East	Fatal	802	781	776	762	569	559	531	474	470	6.0
	KSI	12,069	10,014	9,415	8,769	6,829	6,809	6,273	6,305	6,160	79.1
	Total	45,503	44,990	47,032	46,198	41,860	42,727	41,895	43,976	43,408	557.5
London	Fatal	539	446	460	409	368	316	286	270	214	3.1
	KSI	8,230	9,478	9,344	8,923	7,878	7,233	6,419	6,195	6,510	93.4
	Total	54,156	50,114	52,779	51,995	46,578	46,417	45,927	45,837	44,995	645.8
South West	Fatal	484	462	521	468	460	385	310	336	358	7.5
	KSI	8,047	6,134	5,781	5,424	4,555	4,153	3,916	3,608	3,455	72.0
	Total	26,352	25,444	25,246	25,034	22,515	22,302	22,728	23,413	23,500	490.0
England	Fatal	4,698	4,283	4,587	4,423	3,854	3,549	3,228	3,077	2,995	6.1
	KSI	67,388	58,215	57,813	55,821	47,404	45,297	41,790	42,403	41,676	85.6
	Total	280,382	281,987	297,952	297,476	270,842	271,759	269,287	277,501	273,373	561.3
Wales	Fatal	259	226	233	249	227	220	187	210	218	7.5
	KSI	3,855	3,127	3,191	3,037	2,638	2,537	2,189	2,208	2,133	73.2
	Total	14,395	15,164	16,165	16,432	15,074	14,732	14,331	15,105	14,950	513.2
Scotland	Fatal	641	543	553	545	487	460	399	363	408	7.9
	KSI	8,887	7,177	7,527	6,800	6,131	5,640	4,844	5,570	5,335	103.9
	Total	27,134	25,056	27,475	27,233	25,353	24,182	22,402	22,583	22,183	432.2
Great Britain	Fatal	5,598	5,052	5,373	5,217	4,568	4,229	3,814	3,650	3,621	6.4
	KSI	80,130	68,519	68,531	65,658	56,173	53,474	48,823	50,181	49,144	86.6
	Total	321,912	322,207	341,592	341,141	311,269	310,673	306,020	315,189	310,506	547.1
Northern Ireland	Fatal	196	178	181	185	185	150	143	157	144	8.8
	KSI	2,362	2,147	2,195	2,178	1,833	1,991	1,725	1,805	1,676	102.1
	Total	8,204	10,967	11,611	11,761	10,314	11,264	11,100	12,094	11,725	714.2
United Kingdom	Fatal	5,794	5,230	5,554	5,402	4,753	4,379	3,957	3,807	3,765	6.4
	KSI	82,492	70,666	70,726	67,836	58,006	55,465	50,548	51,986	50,820	87.0
	Total	330,116	333,174	353,203	352,902	321,583	321,937	317,120	327,283	322,231	551.8

1 1994 population data used. 1995 data not yet available.

2 Number of casualties: by county and road user type: 1995

	Children (0-15)	Adults (16-59)	Elderly (60+)	All[1] casualties	Pedest- rians	Pedal cyclists	Motor cyclists	Car occupants	Other[2] road users
Avon	512	3,135	417	4,072	627	358	423	2,401	263
Bedfordshire	383	2,188	220	2,791	342	189	200	1,891	169
Berkshire	503	2,972	305	3,960	412	410	324	2,655	159
Buckinghamshire	431	2,810	278	3,664	338	240	268	2,652	166
Cambridgeshire	529	3,384	377	4,361	337	650	365	2,760	249
Cheshire	812	5,229	607	6,648	614	471	404	4,664	495
Cleveland	455	1,759	220	2,434	487	217	64	1,543	123
Cornwall	299	1,893	285	2,477	303	155	214	1,673	132
Cumbria	397	1,978	313	2,688	322	210	194	1,765	197
Derbyshire	662	3,778	437	5,041	622	339	441	3,292	347
Devon	651	3,790	569	5,030	697	426	579	3,054	274
Dorset	418	2,640	504	3,562	324	310	309	2,390	229
Durham	480	2,107	294	2,881	444	148	118	1,923	248
East Sussex	527	2,820	578	3,925	647	321	330	2,364	263
Essex	1,105	6,736	849	9,116	1,055	689	717	6,132	523
Gloucestershire	335	1,998	307	2,640	271	237	269	1,711	152
Greater London	5,218	32,459	3,956	44,995	9,373	4,513	5,443	22,204	3,462
Greater Manchester	2,717	12,138	1,334	16,189	2,960	1,220	601	10,274	1,134
Hampshire	1,178	6,949	875	9,002	962	1,045	861	5,589	545
Hereford & Worcester	480	2,696	403	3,579	396	284	322	2,341	236
Hertfordshire	766	5,011	553	6,398	569	420	459	4,613	337
Humberside	821	3,425	505	4,751	765	728	469	2,467	322
Isle of Wight	88	441	113	642	95	73	77	347	50
Kent	1,076	5,855	751	7,810	1,011	575	818	5,019	387
Lancashire	1,462	6,494	947	8,922	1,384	670	529	5,720	619
Leicestershire	679	3,559	483	4,765	692	404	330	3,038	301
Lincolnshire	473	2,782	426	3,681	348	304	294	2,523	212
Merseyside	1,515	6,699	959	9,173	1,472	585	305	6,063	748
Norfolk	464	2,778	510	3,880	375	309	366	2,635	195
Northamptonshire	372	2,334	256	2,965	370	200	201	2,029	165
Northumberland	211	1,100	185	1,496	155	88	72	1,041	140
North Yorkshire	552	3,522	585	4,679	462	340	465	3,075	337
Nottinghamshire	915	4,065	516	5,879	875	461	462	3,581	500
Oxfordshire	342	2,351	284	3,080	265	351	293	1,963	208
Shropshire	272	1,720	246	2,238	213	149	148	1,557	171
Somerset	316	1,845	311	2,485	224	187	189	1,762	123
South Yorkshire	1,035	4,199	678	5,926	1,108	377	286	3,578	577
Staffordshire	857	4,830	621	6,611	746	467	451	4,451	496
Suffolk	372	2,000	328	2,707	303	282	270	1,703	149
Surrey	702	5,686	724	7,569	637	596	619	5,370	347
Tyne & Wear	864	3,317	522	4,703	1,056	339	107	2,803	398
Warwickshire	324	2,347	284	3,083	268	230	295	2,105	185
West Midlands	2,209	8,580	1,173	11,962	2,504	905	599	7,300	654
West Sussex	467	2,792	497	3,756	360	407	318	2,467	204
West Yorkshire	1,957	8,736	1,230	11,923	2,239	706	549	7,554	875
Wiltshire	394	2,496	331	3,234	324	261	280	2,140	229
England	37,597	202,423	27,146	273,373	40,353	22,846	21,697	170,182	18,295
Wales	2,257	10,968	1,725	14,950	2,042	745	812	10,384	967
Scotland	3,934	15,680	2,569	22,183	4,634	1,322	971	13,426	1,830
Great Britain	43,788	229,071	31,440	310,506	47,029	24,913	23,480	193,992	21,092
Northern Ireland	1,719	9,068	938	11,725	1,229	385	248	8,843	1,020
United Kingdom	45,507	238,139	32,378	322,231	48,258	25,298	23,728	202,835	22,112

1 Includes age not reported.
2 Includes road user type not reported.

3 Number of casualties: by county and road user type: 1981-85 average[1]

	Children (0-15)	Adults (16-59)	Older adults (60+)	All[2] casualties	Pedest-rians	Pedal cyclists	Motor cyclists	Car occupants	Other[3] road users
Avon	616	3,520	447	4,584	777	402	1,399	1,768	238
Bedfordshire	502	2,480	252	3,235	495	299	628	1,552	262
Berkshire	573	3,232	333	4,243	567	449	904	2,167	157
Buckinghamshire	464	2,713	283	3,504	409	287	700	1,940	168
Cambridgeshire	489	3,095	397	3,981	345	646	923	1,834	233
Cheshire	803	3,789	490	5,095	711	593	1,126	2,324	341
Cleveland	587	1,853	231	2,671	682	274	515	1,016	185
Cornwall	359	2,079	253	2,691	339	151	756	1,301	144
Cumbria	441	2,068	297	2,806	444	216	606	1,383	157
Derbyshire	715	3,505	439	4,933	808	405	1,207	2,098	415
Devon	769	4,333	624	5,726	845	400	1,654	2,526	302
Dorset	461	2,745	471	3,677	487	396	959	1,647	188
Durham	450	1,806	221	2,476	510	140	412	1,216	198
East Sussex	535	2,722	655	3,911	725	287	830	1,842	227
Essex	1,344	7,165	947	9,474	1,212	803	1,845	5,003	611
Gloucestershire	419	2,549	308	3,276	378	348	926	1,465	160
Greater London	7,106	37,831	5,855	54,156	13,081	4,739	9,957	21,778	4,601
Greater Manchester	2,946	9,320	1,431	13,699	3,931	1,376	2,284	5,186	922
Hampshire	1,276	7,151	881	9,308	1,159	1,182	2,530	3,981	456
Hereford & Worcester	491	2,895	384	3,770	461	370	847	1,909	183
Hertfordshire	784	4,401	485	5,729	738	511	1,173	3,003	304
Humberside	842	3,601	491	4,934	821	727	1,377	1,620	388
Isle of Wight	107	481	74	662	107	61	206	260	28
Kent	1,251	6,769	848	8,867	1,246	744	2,291	4,139	447
Lancashire	1,399	5,155	906	7,460	1,683	666	1,458	3,188	466
Leicestershire	752	3,657	415	4,825	827	507	1,117	2,124	249
Lincolnshire	501	2,866	382	3,749	365	381	852	1,929	221
Merseyside	1,632	4,718	875	7,225	2,066	583	1,009	2,926	642
Norfolk	551	3,195	495	4,241	483	456	1,063	1,999	240
Northamptonshire	499	2,818	334	3,652	449	240	779	1,913	271
Northumberland	215	1,142	159	1,516	192	95	270	828	131
North Yorkshire	568	3,349	496	4,413	531	420	1,030	2,150	283
Nottinghamshire	987	4,364	570	5,920	1,111	609	1,362	2,381	458
Oxfordshire	389	2,677	297	3,424	362	382	798	1,663	219
Shropshire	297	1,767	211	2,275	252	185	473	1,237	129
Somerset	299	1,875	276	2,450	267	222	640	1,204	117
South Yorkshire	1,108	4,121	685	5,914	1,475	354	1,069	2,308	708
Staffordshire	1,038	4,972	518	6,528	983	558	1,388	3,167	432
Suffolk	479	2,762	385	3,627	397	389	961	1,696	183
Surrey	921	5,844	779	7,640	808	838	1,764	3,918	312
Tyne & Wear	1,028	2,906	509	4,443	1,491	334	650	1,568	400
Warwickshire	400	2,179	261	2,839	339	295	606	1,446	154
West Midlands	2,714	8,345	1,227	12,286	3,596	1,064	1,993	4,812	820
West Sussex	498	2,919	527	3,943	440	464	907	1,953	180
West Yorkshire	2,039	7,531	1,084	10,654	2,728	722	2,048	4,386	770
Wiltshire	491	3,080	377	3,948	392	358	887	2,056	256
England	43,133	204,343	28,867	280,382	52,515	25,927	59,179	123,806	18,956
Wales	2,320	10,500	1,576	14,395	2,666	857	2,566	7,211	1,094
Scotland	4,881	19,157	3,097	27,134	6,560	1,607	3,446	12,924	2,598
Great Britain	50,334	234,000	33,540	321,912	61,741	28,391	65,191	143,941	22,647
Northern Ireland[4]	1,516	5,954	731	8,204	1,648	399	765	5,398	
United Kingdom[4]	51,850	239,954	34,271	330,115	63,389	28,791	65,956	171,986	

1 Figures have been rounded so there may be an apparent slight discrepancy between the sum of the constituent items and the total as shown.
2 Includes age not reported.
3 Includes road user type not reported.
4 It is not possible to give separate casualty figures for car occupants and other road users for Northern Ireland for these years.

4 Total casualty rates[1]: by county and road user type: 1995

Rate per 100,000 population

	Children (0-15)	Adults (16-59)	Elderly (60+)	All[2] casualties	Pedest-rians	Pedal cyclists	Motor cyclists	Car occupants	Other[3] road users
Avon	267	539	203	416	64	37	43	245	27
Bedfordshire	314	665	239	514	63	35	37	348	31
Berkshire	306	623	238	515	54	53	42	345	21
Buckinghamshire	298	696	252	557	51	36	41	403	25
Cambridgeshire	373	811	295	635	49	95	53	402	36
Cheshire	398	906	312	681	63	48	41	478	51
Cleveland	357	541	204	435	87	39	11	275	22
Cornwall	322	715	234	516	63	32	45	349	28
Cumbria	415	702	278	548	66	43	40	360	40
Derbyshire	346	674	216	528	65	36	46	345	36
Devon	326	645	213	478	66	40	55	290	26
Dorset	345	722	271	529	48	46	46	355	34
Durham	386	593	229	474	73	24	19	316	41
East Sussex	399	710	293	540	89	44	45	325	36
Essex	348	731	256	581	67	44	46	391	33
Gloucestershire	306	627	253	480	49	43	49	311	28
Greater London	368	753	319	646	135	65	78	319	50
Greater Manchester	482	802	266	628	115	47	23	399	44
Hampshire	360	727	272	561	60	65	54	348	34
Hereford & Worcester	338	662	268	511	57	41	46	334	34
Hertfordshire	367	835	281	636	57	42	46	459	34
Humberside	439	666	269	534	86	82	53	277	36
Isle of Wight	385	673	312	515	76	59	62	278	40
Kent	337	653	228	505	65	37	53	325	25
Lancashire	488	795	308	627	97	47	37	402	43
Leicestershire	350	651	274	520	75	44	36	331	33
Lincolnshire	404	811	293	608	57	50	49	417	35
Merseyside	493	814	315	639	103	41	21	423	52
Norfolk	321	640	268	505	49	40	48	343	25
Northamptonshire	286	660	230	498	62	34	34	341	28
Northumberland	344	618	271	486	50	29	23	338	45
North Yorkshire	396	839	351	644	64	47	64	423	46
Nottinghamshire	435	666	245	570	85	45	45	347	49
Oxfordshire	282	651	264	522	45	59	50	333	35
Shropshire	316	705	285	537	51	36	36	374	41
Somerset	332	694	266	520	47	39	40	369	26
South Yorkshire	390	546	249	454	85	29	22	274	44
Staffordshire	396	767	299	627	71	44	43	422	47
Suffolk	278	543	223	417	47	43	42	262	23
Surrey	346	919	329	727	61	57	59	516	33
Tyne & Wear	372	503	216	415	93	30	9	247	35
Warwickshire	329	794	278	621	54	46	59	424	37
West Midlands	382	565	221	455	95	34	23	278	25
West Sussex	340	702	265	520	50	56	44	342	28
West Yorkshire	432	705	299	567	106	34	26	359	42
Wiltshire	324	718	283	552	55	45	48	365	39
England	376	706	271	561	83	47	45	349	38
Wales	372	663	264	513	70	26	28	356	33
Scotland	379	512	249	432	90	26	19	262	36
Great Britain	376	686	268	547	83	44	41	342	37
Northern Ireland	410	961	337	714	75	23	15	539	62
United Kingdom	377	694	270	552	83	43	41	347	38

1 Based on mid year 1994 population estimates.
2 Includes age not reported.
3 Includes road user type not reported.

5 Casualty indicators: by county and road user type: 1995

	Percentage of all casualties who are:							Other[2]
	Children[1] (0-15)	Adults[1] (16-59)	Elderly[1] (60+)	Pedest-rians	Pedal cyclists	Motor cyclists	Car occupants	road users
Avon	12.6	77.1	10.3	15.4	8.8	10.4	59.0	6.5
Bedfordshire	13.7	78.4	7.9	12.3	6.8	7.2	67.8	6.1
Berkshire	13.3	78.6	8.1	10.4	10.4	8.2	67.0	4.0
Buckinghamshire	12.2	79.9	7.9	9.2	6.6	7.3	72.4	4.5
Cambridgeshire	12.3	78.9	8.8	7.7	14.9	8.4	63.3	5.7
Cheshire	12.2	78.7	9.1	9.2	7.1	6.1	70.2	7.4
Cleveland	18.7	72.3	9.0	20.0	8.9	2.6	63.4	5.1
Cornwall	12.1	76.4	11.5	12.2	6.3	8.6	67.5	5.3
Cumbria	14.8	73.6	11.6	12.0	7.8	7.2	65.7	7.3
Derbyshire	13.6	77.5	9.0	12.3	6.7	8.7	65.3	6.9
Devon	13.0	75.6	11.4	13.9	8.5	11.5	60.7	5.4
Dorset	11.7	74.1	14.1	9.1	8.7	8.7	67.1	6.4
Durham	16.7	73.1	10.2	15.4	5.1	4.1	66.7	8.6
East Sussex	13.4	71.8	14.7	16.5	8.2	8.4	60.2	6.7
Essex	12.7	77.5	9.8	11.6	7.6	7.9	67.3	5.7
Gloucestershire	12.7	75.7	11.6	10.3	9.0	10.2	64.8	5.8
Greater London	12.5	78.0	9.5	20.8	10.0	12.1	49.3	7.7
Greater Manchester	16.8	75.0	8.2	18.3	7.5	3.7	63.5	7.0
Hampshire	13.1	77.2	9.7	10.7	11.6	9.6	62.1	6.1
Hereford & Worcester	13.4	75.3	11.3	11.1	7.9	9.0	65.4	6.6
Hertfordshire	12.1	79.2	8.7	8.9	6.6	7.2	72.1	5.3
Humberside	17.3	72.1	10.6	16.1	15.3	9.9	51.9	6.8
Isle of Wight	13.7	68.7	17.6	14.8	11.4	12.0	54.0	7.8
Kent	14.0	76.2	9.8	12.9	7.4	10.5	64.3	5.0
Lancashire	16.4	72.9	10.6	15.5	7.5	5.9	64.1	6.9
Leicestershire	14.4	75.4	10.2	14.5	8.5	6.9	63.8	6.3
Lincolnshire	12.8	75.6	11.6	9.5	8.3	8.0	68.5	5.8
Merseyside	16.5	73.0	10.5	16.0	6.4	3.3	66.1	8.2
Norfolk	12.4	74.0	13.6	9.7	8.0	9.4	67.9	5.0
Northamptonshire	12.6	78.8	8.6	12.5	6.7	6.8	68.4	5.6
Northumberland	14.1	73.5	12.4	10.4	5.9	4.8	69.6	9.4
North Yorkshire	11.8	75.6	12.6	9.9	7.3	9.9	65.7	7.2
Nottinghamshire	16.6	74.0	9.4	14.9	7.8	7.9	60.9	8.5
Oxfordshire	11.5	79.0	9.5	8.6	11.4	9.5	63.7	6.8
Shropshire	12.2	76.9	11.0	9.5	6.7	6.6	69.6	7.6
Somerset	12.8	74.6	12.6	9.0	7.5	7.6	70.9	4.9
South Yorkshire	17.5	71.0	11.5	18.7	6.4	4.8	60.4	9.7
Staffordshire	13.6	76.6	9.8	11.3	7.1	6.8	67.3	7.5
Suffolk	13.8	74.1	12.1	11.2	10.4	10.0	62.9	5.5
Surrey	9.9	79.9	10.2	8.4	7.9	8.2	70.9	4.6
Tyne & Wear	18.4	70.5	11.1	22.5	7.2	2.3	59.6	8.5
Warwickshire	11.0	79.4	9.6	8.7	7.5	9.6	68.3	6.0
West Midlands	18.5	71.7	9.8	20.9	7.6	5.0	61.0	5.5
West Sussex	12.4	74.3	13.2	9.6	10.8	8.5	65.7	5.4
West Yorkshire	16.4	73.3	10.3	18.8	5.9	4.6	63.4	7.3
Wiltshire	12.2	77.5	10.3	10.0	8.1	8.7	66.2	7.1
England	14.1	75.8	10.2	14.8	8.4	7.9	62.3	6.7
Wales	15.1	73.4	11.5	13.7	5.0	5.4	69.5	6.5
Scotland	17.7	70.7	11.6	20.9	6.0	4.4	60.5	8.2
Great Britain	14.4	75.3	10.3	15.1	8.0	7.6	62.5	6.8
Northern Ireland	14.7	77.3	8.0	10.5	3.3	2.1	75.4	8.7
United Kingdom	14.4	75.4	10.2	15.0	7.9	7.4	62.9	6.9

1 Percentage of casualties of known age.
2 Includes road user type not reported.

6 Casualty changes: by county and severity: 1981-85 average, 1995

Number of casualties

	Fatal and serious casualties			Total casualties		
	1981-85 average	1995	Percentage change	1981-85 average	1995	Percentage change
Avon	1,356	559	-58.8	4,584	4,072	-11.2
Bedfordshire	714	406	-43.2	3,235	2,791	-13.7
Berkshire	1,095	330	-69.9	4,243	3,960	-6.7
Buckinghamshire	1,031	398	-61.4	3,504	3,664	4.6
Cambridgeshire	1,087	732	-32.6	3,981	4,361	9.6
Cheshire	916	1,257	37.2	5,095	6,648	30.5
Cleveland	486	224	-53.9	2,671	2,434	-8.9
Cornwall	858	363	-57.7	2,691	2,477	-7.9
Cumbria	829	588	-29.1	2,806	2,688	-4.2
Derbyshire	1,222	823	-32.6	4,933	5,041	2.2
Devon	1,897	698	-63.2	5,726	5,030	-12.2
Dorset	940	478	-49.2	3,677	3,562	-3.1
Durham	703	397	-43.5	2,476	2,881	16.3
East Sussex	989	581	-41.2	3,911	3,925	0.3
Essex	2,398	1,461	-39.1	9,474	9,116	-3.8
Gloucestershire	1,166	396	-66.0	3,276	2,640	-19.4
Greater London[1]	8,230 (9,175)	6,510	-20.9	54,156	44,995	-16.9
Greater Manchester	2,362	1,334	-43.5	13,699	16,189	18.2
Hampshire	2,755	1,381	-49.9	9,308	9,002	-3.3
Hereford & Worcester	1,071	796	-25.7	3,770	3,579	-5.1
Hertfordshire	1,388	1,025	-26.1	5,729	6,398	11.7
Humberside	1,129	890	-21.1	4,934	4,751	-3.7
Isle of Wight	184	108	-41.3	662	642	-3.0
Kent	2,385	1,400	-41.3	8,867	7,810	-11.9
Lancashire	1,704	1,696	-0.5	7,460	8,922	19.6
Leicestershire	1,226	627	-48.9	4,825	4,765	-1.2
Lincolnshire	1,074	729	-32.1	3,749	3,681	-1.8
Merseyside	1,237	823	-33.5	7,225	9,173	27.0
Norfolk	1,524	942	-38.2	4,241	3,880	-8.5
Northamptonshire	1,328	805	-39.4	3,652	2,965	-18.8
Northumberland	400	261	-34.7	1,516	1,496	-1.3
North Yorkshire	1,835	1,186	-35.4	4,413	4,679	6.0
Nottinghamshire	1,540	1,156	-24.9	5,920	5,879	-0.7
Oxfordshire	1,067	395	-63.0	3,424	3,080	-10.0
Shropshire	833	556	-33.3	2,275	2,238	-1.6
Somerset	811	407	-49.8	2,450	2,485	1.4
South Yorkshire	1,320	746	-43.5	5,914	5,926	0.2
Staffordshire	1,442	639	-55.7	6,528	6,611	1.3
Suffolk	1,170	474	-59.5	3,627	2,707	-25.4
Surrey	1,641	959	-41.6	7,640	7,569	-0.9
Tyne & Wear	1,048	634	-39.5	4,443	4,703	5.8
Warwickshire	1,059	665	-37.2	2,839	3,083	8.6
West Midlands	3,452	2,057	-40.4	12,286	11,962	-2.6
West Sussex	922	608	-34.0	3,943	3,756	-4.8
West Yorkshire	2,547	1,622	-36.3	10,654	11,923	11.9
Wiltshire	1,019	554	-45.6	3,948	3,234	-18.1
England	67,388	41,676	-38.2	280,382	273,373	-2.5
Wales	3,855	2,133	-44.7	14,395	14,950	3.9
Scotland	8,887	5,335	-40.0	27,134	22,183	-18.2
Great Britain	80,130	49,144	-38.7	321,912	310,506	-3.5
Northern Ireland	2,362	1,676	-29.0	8,204	11,725	42.9
United Kingdom	82,492	50,820	-38.4	330,116	322,231	-2.4

1 In September 1984 the Metropolitan Police implemented revised standards in the assessment of serious casualties.
  Figures in brackets estimate casualty totals under standards prevailing since 1984. See preface.

7 Number of casualties: by road class, Government Office Region[1] and severity: 1995

Number of casualties

		Motorways	Built-Up				Non Built-Up				All Roads[2]
			Trunk	Principle	Other	Total	Trunk	Principle	Other	Total	
North East	Fatal	7	1	23	49	73	12	43	17	72	152
	KSI	19	9	299	621	929	104	256	208	568	1,516
	Total	176	116	2,588	5,231	7,935	893	1,462	1,048	3,403	11,514
North West	Fatal	22	5	104	85	194	37	61	44	142	358
	KSI	209	82	1,262	1,911	3,255	314	629	468	1,411	4,875
	Total	1,975	682	11,446	14,164	26,292	1,520	2,631	2,029	6,180	34,447
Merseyside	Fatal	4	2	22	22	46	4	2	4	10	60
	KSI	18	18	305	399	722	29	26	28	83	823
	Total	246	307	3,284	4,659	8,250	255	183	239	677	9,173
North West/Merseyside	Fatal	26	7	126	107	240	41	63	48	152	418
	KSI	227	100	1,567	2,310	3,977	343	655	496	1,494	5,698
	Total	2,221	989	14,730	18,823	34,542	1,775	2,814	2,268	6,857	43,620
Yorkshire/Humberside	Fatal	19	7	64	104	175	45	66	40	151	345
	KSI	117	74	1,002	1,693	2,769	381	607	570	1,558	4,444
	Total	895	614	7,244	12,031	19,889	1,512	2,645	2,338	6,495	27,279
East Midlands	Fatal	9	7	47	74	128	70	95	76	241	378
	KSI	106	144	701	1,250	2,095	477	762	700	1,939	4,140
	Total	659	967	4,497	7,871	13,335	2,140	3,297	2,900	8,337	22,331
West Midlands	Fatal	18	8	63	60	131	36	60	41	137	286
	KSI	195	122	1,102	1,807	3,031	329	568	590	1,487	4,713
	Total	1,267	709	7,567	11,330	19,606	1,676	2,453	2,471	6,600	27,473
Eastern	Fatal	20	3	30	41	74	106	86	88	280	374
	KSI	173	82	714	1,487	2,283	660	827	1,097	2,584	5,040
	Total	1,598	557	5,229	9,982	15,768	3,111	4,008	4,767	11,886	29,253
South East	Fatal	27	6	68	84	158	56	135	94	285	470
	KSI	316	100	1,183	1,878	3,161	382	1,210	1,091	2,683	6,160
	Total	2,779	781	9,659	14,723	25,163	2,419	6,631	6,414	15,464	43,408
London	Fatal	9	21	102	74	197	4	4	0	8	214
	KSI	80	595	3,191	2,424	6,210	150	41	29	220	6,510
	Total	611	4,523	22,014	16,555	43,092	934	191	166	1,291	44,995
South West	Fatal	31	1	54	59	114	33	106	71	210	358
	KSI	133	33	542	1,020	1,595	268	761	695	1,724	3,455
	Total	785	328	4,421	8,124	12,873	1,620	4,275	3,933	9,828	23,500
England	Fatal	166	61	577	652	1,290	403	658	475	1,536	2,995
	KSI	1,366	1,259	10,301	14,490	26,050	3,094	5,687	5,476	14,257	41,676
	Total	10,991	9,584	77,949	104,670	192,203	16,080	27,776	26,305	70,161	273,373
Wales	Fatal	4	7	31	42	80	59	52	23	134	218
	KSI	38	70	310	642	1,022	421	349	303	1,073	2,133
	Total	323	544	2,629	6,060	9,233	1,840	1,905	1,649	5,394	14,950
Scotland	Fatal	10	6	47	74	127	112	104	55	271	408
	KSI	109	103	943	1,809	2,855	787	914	670	2,371	5,335
	Total	537	560	4,441	8,533	13,534	2,433	3,230	2,449	8,112	22,183
Great Britain	Fatal	180	74	655	768	1,497	574	814	553	1,941	3,621
	KSI	1,513	1,432	11,554	16,941	29,927	4,302	6,950	6,449	17,701	49,144
	Total	11,851	10,688	85,019	119,263	214,970	20,353	32,911	30,403	83,667	310,506

1 Casualty data by road class are not available for Northern Ireland.
2 Includes speed limit not reported.

8 Casualty rates per 100 million vehicle kilometres: by road class, Government Office Region[1] and severity: 1993-1995 average

Rate per 100 million vehicle kilometres

			A Roads					
			Built-Up		Non Built-Up			All major roads[2]
		Motorways	Trunk	Principle	Trunk	Principle	All A Roads	
North East	Fatal	0.7	0.5	1.1	0.6	1.1	0.9	0.9
	KSI	2.5	10.1	13.7	4.0	8.0	8.2	7.7
	Total	21.0	151.7	106.5	31.2	47.1	59.2	55.7
North West	Fatal	0.3	1.0	1.1	1.1	1.4	1.2	0.8
	KSI	2.1	14.7	14.6	9.0	12.0	12.7	8.6
	Total	18.4	116.8	131.1	43.5	58.7	93.7	64.7
Merseyside	Fatal	0.3	0.9	1.7	1.0	1.6	1.5	1.2
	KSI	2.2	9.5	18.7	6.9	10.2	15.2	12.1
	Total	29.3	155.7	206.2	60.6	81.1	167.1	134.3
North West/Merseyside	Fatal	0.3	0.9	1.2	1.1	1.4	1.2	0.9
	KSI	2.1	13.3	15.3	8.8	11.9	13.1	9.0
	Total	19.2	127.8	143.9	45.3	59.9	103.5	72.4
Yorkshire/Humberside	Fatal	0.3	1.2	1.3	0.8	1.7	1.2	1.0
	KSI	1.8	11.7	15.4	8.4	14.9	13.1	10.3
	Total	16.8	91.6	111.3	33.1	61.7	74.7	60.6
East Midlands	Fatal	0.2	1.2	1.2	1.0	1.6	1.3	1.1
	KSI	2.6	13.0	17.5	7.4	13.7	12.1	10.2
	Total	17.1	90.5	117.5	34.1	60.4	65.1	55.3
West Midlands	Fatal	0.3	1.0	1.2	1.2	1.6	1.3	0.9
	KSI	2.5	13.6	17.5	9.3	12.5	13.8	9.8
	Total	14.8	95.4	114.1	41.8	53.9	78.0	55.5
Eastern	Fatal	0.3	0.7	0.8	0.9	1.3	1.0	0.8
	KSI	2.6	13.7	14.9	6.4	11.7	10.2	8.5
	Total	21.1	99.9	108.0	30.7	55.0	56.9	48.9
South East	Fatal	0.2	1.7	0.8	0.7	1.1	0.9	0.7
	KSI	1.9	18.9	12.7	5.1	9.3	9.5	6.8
	Total	16.1	144.0	97.6	30.4	52.6	62.9	46.5
London	Fatal	0.3	1.0	1.2	0.3	0.8	1.0	0.9
	KSI	4.3	19.0	29.1	5.8	11.1	23.2	21.3
	Total	32.9	143.7	207.6	36.8	69.8	166.2	152.5
South West	Fatal	0.4	0.4	0.8	0.8	1.4	1.0	0.9
	KSI	2.0	10.5	9.8	5.3	10.4	8.8	7.2
	Total	12.8	99.8	77.2	29.5	53.7	54.3	44.9
England	Fatal	0.3	1.0	1.1	0.9	1.3	1.1	0.9
	KSI	2.2	15.7	17.1	6.7	11.3	12.3	9.6
	Total	17.5	121.4	128.8	33.7	55.3	79.0	62.4
Wales	Fatal	0.2	0.9	1.0	1.2	1.4	1.2	1.0
	KSI	1.5	9.5	11.3	9.2	11.2	10.4	9.0
	Total	13.5	67.5	91.1	42.8	57.4	61.5	54.3
Scotland	Fatal	0.4	0.9	0.8	1.4	1.5	1.3	1.1
	KSI	3.1	14.0	15.8	10.3	14.3	13.2	11.7
	Total	14.1	66.3	80.2	33.6	50.3	52.9	47.0
Great Britain	Fatal	0.3	1.0	1.0	0.9	1.4	1.1	0.9
	KSI	2.3	15.0	16.7	7.3	11.6	12.3	9.7
	Total	17.2	112.0	123.3	34.3	54.9	75.3	60.6

1 Casualty and traffic data by road class are not available for Northern Ireland.
2 Includes road class and type not reported.

9 Accident rates per 100 million vehicle kilometres: by road class, Government Office Region[1] and severity: 1993-1995 average

Rate per 100 million vehicle kilometres

			A Roads					
			Built-Up		Non Built-Up			All major
		Motorways	Trunk	Principle	Trunk	Principle	All A Roads	roads[2]
North East	Fatal	0.6	0.5	1.1	0.5	1.0	0.8	0.8
	Fatal or serious	1.8	9.7	12.6	3.1	6.0	6.9	6.4
	All severities	12.7	111.6	79.7	18.0	28.1	39.8	37.4
North West	Fatal	0.2	0.9	1.0	1.0	1.3	1.1	0.7
	Fatal or serious	1.5	12.9	13.1	6.3	9.0	10.6	7.1
	All severities	11.2	82.2	95.1	25.8	36.8	65.2	44.4
Merseyside	Fatal	0.3	0.9	1.6	1.0	1.5	1.4	1.1
	Fatal or serious	1.8	8.4	16.9	5.1	7.0	13.4	10.6
	All severities	17.9	102.0	141.1	33.3	46.7	111.8	89.5
North West/Merseyside	Fatal	0.2	0.9	1.1	1.0	1.3	1.1	0.8
	Fatal or serious	1.6	11.6	13.7	6.2	8.9	11.0	7.5
	All severities	11.7	87.9	102.9	26.6	37.3	71.4	49.4
Yorkshire/Humberside	Fatal	0.3	1.1	1.2	0.7	1.4	1.1	0.9
	Fatal or serious	1.4	10.2	13.6	5.5	10.4	10.3	8.1
	All severities	10.6	68.4	83.6	19.2	37.0	51.9	41.9
East Midlands	Fatal	0.2	1.2	1.1	0.9	1.4	1.1	0.9
	Fatal or serious	1.9	11.7	15.5	5.5	10.2	9.7	8.1
	All severities	10.0	67.4	88.6	20.3	37.6	44.4	37.4
West Midlands	Fatal	0.2	1.0	1.1	1.1	1.3	1.1	0.8
	Fatal or serious	1.8	11.4	15.1	6.7	9.4	11.2	7.9
	All severities	8.9	69.4	85.5	26.2	35.3	55.6	39.0
Eastern	Fatal	0.3	0.7	0.8	0.8	1.1	0.9	0.7
	Fatal or serious	2.0	12.1	13.5	4.8	8.9	8.2	6.8
	All severities	13.1	73.9	84.2	19.0	35.6	39.7	33.8
South East	Fatal	0.1	1.5	0.8	0.6	1.0	0.8	0.6
	Fatal or serious	1.4	15.8	11.6	3.9	7.3	7.9	5.6
	All severities	9.9	106.0	76.7	19.1	34.4	45.2	32.8
London	Fatal	0.2	0.9	1.2	0.3	0.7	1.0	0.9
	Fatal or serious	3.4	16.5	26.8	4.7	9.1	21.1	19.2
	All severities	23.9	116.2	176.8	26.8	52.9	139.6	127.6
South West	Fatal	0.3	0.4	0.7	0.7	1.2	0.9	0.7
	Fatal or serious	1.3	9.3	8.7	3.8	7.8	7.0	5.7
	All severities	7.7	76.0	61.3	18.4	34.0	38.1	31.2
England	Fatal	0.2	1.0	1.0	0.8	1.2	1.0	0.8
	Fatal or serious	1.7	13.6	15.4	4.9	8.5	10.2	7.9
	All severities	10.8	93.1	100.7	20.7	35.2	57.6	45.0
Wales	Fatal	0.2	0.8	0.9	0.9	1.3	1.0	0.9
	Fatal or serious	1.2	7.9	9.4	6.1	8.0	7.6	6.7
	All severities	8.8	47.0	64.8	24.1	34.1	39.3	34.7
Scotland	Fatal	0.3	0.9	0.8	1.1	1.3	1.1	1.0
	Fatal or serious	2.4	11.7	14.5	6.9	10.4	10.3	9.1
	All severities	8.6	48.1	64.3	20.0	31.9	37.0	32.7
Great Britain	Fatal	0.2	1.0	1.0	0.8	1.2	1.0	0.8
	Fatal or serious	1.7	13.0	15.1	5.2	8.6	10.1	8.0
	All severities	10.6	85.2	96.2	20.9	34.8	54.4	43.4

1 Casualty and traffic data by road class are not available for Northern Ireland.
2 Includes road class and type not reported.

10 Accidents and accident indices[1]: by month, severity and Government Office Region: 1995

Index/number

	Jan	Feb	Mar	Apr	May	Jun	Jul	Aug	Sep	Oct	Nov	Dec	All Accidents
North East													
Fatal or Serious	97	85	94	97	76	92	92	101	113	108	137	110	1,309
All severities	99	95	101	84	91	92	91	95	112	102	125	113	8,309
North West													
Fatal or Serious	93	97	87	96	93	100	97	103	118	108	106	102	4,146
All severities	98	95	98	86	95	98	96	98	112	108	109	107	24,573
Merseyside													
Fatal or Serious	92	114	124	91	90	113	67	88	116	88	86	132	733
All severities	92	102	106	95	101	87	90	92	108	105	107	113	6,447
North West/Merseyside													
Fatal or Serious	92	99	92	96	92	102	92	101	118	105	103	107	4,879
All severities	97	97	100	88	96	95	95	96	112	107	109	108	31,020
Yorkshire/Humberside													
Fatal or Serious	96	89	103	90	100	95	107	109	100	101	116	95	3,709
All severities	94	94	105	87	97	94	104	105	105	96	114	105	19,954
East Midlands													
Fatal or Serious	84	89	95	85	90	103	101	101	121	107	113	110	3,466
All severities	96	92	96	85	92	95	98	100	115	106	120	104	15,902
West Midlands													
Fatal or Serious	97	94	106	100	90	109	90	104	99	103	118	90	4,000
All severities	102	99	100	89	97	100	93	96	109	103	112	102	20,030
Eastern													
Fatal or Serious	96	93	100	100	95	103	94	99	103	110	114	92	4,248
All severities	98	93	100	85	92	102	97	99	110	101	120	102	21,074
South East													
Fatal or Serious	90	95	93	88	97	107	107	98	113	103	116	94	5,295
All severities	96	100	96	86	97	100	101	96	109	104	117	99	32,037
London													
Fatal or Serious	85	78	82	103	102	107	107	95	104	115	113	109	5,922
All severities	94	104	103	92	100	102	99	96	110	98	109	95	37,978
South West													
Fatal or Serious	94	103	106	94	101	89	106	106	104	92	107	98	2,843
All severities	87	99	94	85	95	97	106	109	110	102	116	100	17,272
England													
Fatal or Serious	92	91	96	95	95	102	100	101	108	106	113	100	35,671
All severities	96	98	100	87	96	98	99	99	110	102	114	102	203,576
Wales													
Fatal or Serious	88	102	96	99	96	95	105	126	96	103	98	96	1,677
All severities	94	99	95	90	92	95	104	109	109	100	113	99	10,275
Scotland													
Fatal or Serious	97	105	91	98	82	104	103	120	104	101	104	91	4,429
All severities	90	103	100	87	90	99	97	112	107	111	102	101	16,525
Great Britain													
Fatal or Serious	92	93	95	95	94	102	101	104	107	105	112	99	41,777
All severities	95	98	99	87	95	98	99	100	110	103	113	102	230,376
Northern Ireland													
Fatal or Serious	108	103	86	71	107	118	90	97	101	102	109	109	1,271
All severities	96	109	104	85	104	99	84	91	108	110	112	99	6,792
United Kingdom													
Fatal or Serious	93	94	95	95	94	103	100	104	107	105	112	99	43,048
All severities	95	99	100	87	96	98	98	100	110	103	113	102	237,168

1 The base (= 100) is the average number of accidents per day for the region.

11 Accidents on motorways: by carriageway type, junction, number of lanes, Government Office Region[1] and severity: 1995

Number of accidents

		Junction			Non-junction		
		2 lanes	3+ lanes	Circular section of roundabouts	2 lanes	3+ lanes	Total[2]
North East	Fatal or serious	1	0	1	12	0	16
	All severities	21	8	2	49	12	105
North West	Fatal or serious	10	13	0	15	105	166
	All severities	86	92	40	101	722	1,238
Merseyside	Fatal or serious	1	2	3	1	7	15
	All severities	9	3	45	17	65	148
North West/Merseyside	Fatal or serious	11	15	3	16	112	181
	All severities	95	95	85	118	787	1,386
Yorkshire/Humberside	Fatal or serious	3	1	3	11	71	90
	All severities	25	12	75	54	374	560
East Midlands	Fatal or serious	0	8	1	5	63	80
	All severities	7	25	26	9	295	393
West Midlands	Fatal or serious	3	13	1	10	113	145
	All severities	15	71	20	38	580	777
Eastern	Fatal or serious	5	8	0	17	96	138
	All severities	22	83	8	89	676	974
South East	Fatal or serious	7	19	3	27	172	249
	All severities	47	129	61	165	1,185	1,740
London	Fatal or serious	8	16	0	9	30	64
	All severities	69	83	9	71	195	438
of which:							
Inner London	Fatal or serious	0	2	0	1	3	7
	All severities	8	16	5	9	16	61
Outer London	Fatal or serious	8	14	0	8	27	57
	All severities	61	67	4	62	179	377
South West	Fatal or serious	1	1	1	3	67	78
	All severities	22	11	31	37	328	478
England	Fatal or serious	39	81	13	110	724	1,041
	All severities	323	517	317	630	4,432	6,851
Wales	Fatal or serious	3	1	1	11	10	28
	All severities	10	8	18	84	83	209
Scotland	Fatal or serious	5	6	2	41	22	84
	All severities	20	34	12	120	103	332
Great Britain	Fatal or serious	47	88	16	162	756	1,153
	All severities	353	559	347	834	4,618	7,392

1 Accident data by road class are not available for Northern Ireland.
2 Includes slip roads and carriageway type not reported.

12 Accidents on trunk A roads: by carriageway type, junction, number of lanes, Government Office Region[1] and severity: 1995

Number of accidents

	Dual carriageway					Single carriageway							Circular Section of round-about	All Trunk A Roads[6]
	Junction[5]		Non-junction			Junction[5]			Non-junction					
	Number of lanes[2]		Number of lanes[2]			Number of lanes[3]			Number of lanes[3]					
	2	3+	2	3+	All	2[4]	3	4+	2[4]	3	4+	All		
North East														
Fatal or serious	8	2	28	5	43	17	2	1	20	1	0	41	5	89
All severities	110	22	166	37	335	77	8	4	83	4	1	177	100	617
North West														
Fatal or serious	16	15	28	4	63	74	13	10	115	4	6	222	8	294
All severities	184	69	113	16	382	402	43	71	343	9	18	886	96	1,373
Merseyside														
Fatal or serious	9	8	8	1	26	2	0	2	1	0	0	5	3	34
All severities	81	47	41	19	188	49	8	9	21	1	2	90	66	347
North West/Merseyside														
Fatal or serious	25	23	36	5	89	76	13	12	116	4	6	227	11	328
All severities	265	116	154	35	570	451	51	80	364	10	20	976	162	1,720
Yorkshire/Humberside														
Fatal or serious	42	2	66	2	112	80	2	4	85	3	1	175	15	303
All severities	133	11	277	17	438	366	29	36	286	14	12	743	153	1,344
East Midlands														
Fatal or serious	68	5	86	5	164	118	6	17	135	1	9	286	36	486
All severities	204	31	322	20	577	515	29	58	453	8	34	1,097	288	1,967
West Midlands														
Fatal or serious	53	3	54	6	116	88	11	2	104	0	0	205	21	342
All severities	238	26	219	13	496	466	33	3	327	5	0	834	216	1,552
Eastern														
Fatal or serious	71	8	148	17	244	142	10	1	140	4	0	297	29	573
All severities	315	40	647	66	1,068	546	31	5	415	12	0	1,009	290	2,383
South East														
Fatal or serious	54	17	72	23	166	70	3	2	105	7	2	189	33	396
All severities	218	76	456	147	897	377	28	9	381	21	14	830	365	2,115
London														
Fatal or serious	79	119	64	65	327	163	10	31	66	6	8	284	27	640
All severities	607	718	351	441	2,117	1,122	56	249	357	25	69	1,878	311	4,349
of which:														
Inner														
Fatal or serious	23	43	12	16	94	83	0	19	40	4	4	150	4	249
All severities	192	262	72	112	638	580	19	167	165	8	46	985	33	1,671
Outer														
Fatal or serious	56	76	52	49	233	80	10	12	26	2	4	134	23	391
All severities	415	456	279	329	1,479	542	37	82	192	17	23	893	278	2,678
South West														
Fatal or serious	22	3	43	0	68	53	5	0	71	7	0	136	7	212
All severities	96	9	205	15	325	310	27	3	365	24	0	729	167	1,232
England														
Fatal or serious	422	182	597	128	1,329	807	62	70	842	33	26	1,840	184	3,369
All severities	2,186	1,049	2,797	791	6,823	4,230	292	447	3,031	123	150	8,273	2,052	17,279
Wales														
Fatal or serious	28	0	41	2	71	78	8	0	148	15	0	249	3	323
All severities	116	5	203	13	337	391	25	1	515	46	0	978	62	1,382
Scotland														
Fatal or serious	63	4	92	8	167	134	8	3	283	2	9	439	8	619
All severities	176	19	281	29	505	447	11	9	759	8	20	1,254	88	1,857
Great Britain														
Fatal or serious	513	186	730	138	1,567	1,019	78	73	1,273	50	35	2,528	195	4,311
All severities	2,478	1,073	3,281	833	7,665	5,068	328	457	4,305	177	170	10,505	2,202	20,518

1 Accident data by road class are not available for Northern Ireland.
2 Number of lanes in each direction.
3 Number of lanes in both directions.
4 Includes one way streets.
5 Does not include accidents at roundabouts.
6 Includes unknown carriageway type and single track roads.

13 Accidents on principal A roads: by carriageway type, junction, number of lanes, Government Office Region[1] and severity: 1995

Number of accidents

	Dual carriageway					Single carriageway							Circular Section of round about	All Trunk A Roads[6]
	Junction[5]		Non-junction			Junction[5]			Non-junction					
	Number of lanes[2]		Number of lanes[2]			Number of lanes[3]			Number of lanes[3]					
	2	3+	2	3+	All	2[4]	3	4+	2[4]	3	4+	All		
North East														
Fatal or serious	37	11	40	9	97	150	12	7	145	8	4	326	37	463
All severities	273	40	177	35	525	1,020	62	66	630	24	19	1,821	403	2,787
North West														
Fatal or serious	101	46	67	15	229	648	54	76	508	14	21	1,321	29	1,598
All severities	948	401	315	85	1,749	4,480	304	585	1,903	46	114	7,432	393	9,829
Merseyside														
Fatal or serious	39	24	19	9	91	120	3	16	40	3	2	184	16	297
All severities	396	211	130	76	813	858	34	154	255	9	29	1,339	179	2,383
North West/Merseyside														
Fatal or serious	140	70	86	24	320	768	57	92	548	17	23	1,505	45	1,895
All severities	1,344	612	445	161	2,562	5,338	338	739	2,158	55	143	8,771	572	12,212
Yorkshire/Humberside														
Fatal or serious	102	30	74	10	216	523	48	20	422	10	8	1,031	69	1,318
All severities	697	214	360	51	1,322	2,884	207	132	1,671	59	32	4,985	600	6,943
East Midlands														
Fatal or serious	72	11	52	4	139	405	17	91	429	8	37	987	61	1,188
All severities	342	89	227	18	676	2,056	88	408	1,558	24	134	4,268	440	5,397
West Midlands														
Fatal or serious	121	39	108	22	290	531	21	25	454	11	11	1,053	59	1,408
All severities	845	240	418	54	1,557	3,051	114	137	1,671	32	33	5,038	578	7,211
Eastern														
Fatal or serious	66	6	76	4	152	505	26	11	463	9	4	1,018	108	1,288
All severities	431	61	348	37	877	2,610	154	50	1,826	58	22	4,720	1,000	6,678
South East														
Fatal or serious	157	27	129	13	326	755	31	34	712	21	10	1,563	124	2,041
All severities	891	163	695	52	1,801	4,843	219	217	3,051	73	65	8,468	1,456	11,948
London														
Fatal or serious	184	73	92	27	376	1,584	60	288	463	17	55	2,467	87	2,962
All severities	1,290	363	438	117	2,208	10,308	323	1,666	3,005	77	394	15,773	768	18,945
of which:														
Inner														
Fatal or serious	96	51	43	20	210	785	35	217	206	11	39	1,293	28	1,550
All severities	686	237	209	81	1,213	5,316	193	1,292	1,388	46	312	8,547	241	10,105
Outer														
Fatal or serious	88	22	49	7	166	799	25	71	257	6	16	1,174	59	1,412
All severities	604	126	229	36	995	4,992	130	374	1,617	31	82	7,226	527	8,840
South West														
Fatal or serious	35	8	53	10	106	390	21	1	454	13	4	883	61	1,059
All severities	302	66	287	36	691	2,538	112	23	2,076	55	16	4,820	610	6,196
England														
Fatal or serious	914	275	710	123	2,022	5,611	293	569	4,090	114	156	10,833	651	13,622
All severities	6,415	1,848	3,395	561	12,219	34,648	1,617	3,438	17,646	457	858	58,664	6,427	78,317
Wales														
Fatal or serious	30	4	23	3	60	154	16	5	234	5	1	415	24	502
All severities	185	28	108	9	330	1,123	93	42	1,059	28	14	2,359	249	2,956
Scotland														
Fatal or serious	84	21	101	21	227	450	16	67	655	10	38	1,236	41	1,521
All severities	336	111	345	62	854	1,784	58	284	2,039	22	140	4,327	292	5,540
Great Britain														
Fatal or serious	1,028	300	834	147	2,309	6,215	325	641	4,979	129	195	12,484	716	15,645
All severities	6,936	1,987	3,848	632	13,403	37,555	1,768	3,764	20,744	507	1,012	65,350	6,968	86,813

1 Accident data by road class are not available for Northern Ireland.
2 Number of lanes in each direction.
3 Number of lanes in both directions.
4 Includes one way streets.
5 Does not include accidents at roundabouts.
6 Includes unknown carriageway type and single track roads.

14 Accidents: by road class, severity, Government Office Region and county: 1981-85 average, 1994, 1995

Number

	Motorways			Trunk A roads			Principal A roads			All roads		
	Fatal	Fatal or serious	All severities	Fatal	Fatal or serious	All severities	Fatal	Fatal or serious	All severities	Fatal	Fatal or serious	All severities
North East Region												
1981-85	2	15	56	21	133	478	88	813	2,997	205	2,255	8,570
1994	2	13	103	13	106	576	50	482	2,745	127	1,482	8,299
1995	6	16	105	9	89	617	60	463	2,787	135	1,309	8,309
Cleveland[1]												
1981-85	0	0	0	4	19	97	18	174	770	42	423	2,137
1994	0	0	0	4	13	121	11	84	687	32	242	2,015
1995	0	0	0	1	11	138	12	76	679	22	187	1,868
Durham												
1981-85	2	10	35	7	40	110	24	195	585	55	577	1,801
1994	2	8	66	4	22	133	13	87	487	34	312	1,812
1995	5	12	74	2	20	131	18	104	516	47	344	1,984
Northumberland[1]												
1981-85	0	0	0	7	45	163	11	87	280	35	313	1,043
1994	0	0	0	1	46	133	8	69	334	18	236	954
1995	0	0	0	3	35	141	9	68	326	16	206	997
Tyne and Wear												
1981-85	0	5	21	2	29	107	36	357	1,361	73	942	3,588
1994	0	5	37	4	25	189	18	242	1,237	43	692	3,518
1995	1	4	31	3	23	207	21	215	1,266	50	572	3,460
North West/Merseyside Region												
1981-85	34	180	811	61	441	1,607	248	2,403	11,227	558	6,179	28,643
1994	30	199	1,433	47	371	1,849	167	1,886	12,796	393	4,956	31,945
1995	24	181	1,386	44	328	1,720	173	1,895	12,212	387	4,879	31,020
Cheshire												
1981-85	8	44	198	17	92	400	32	277	1,436	83	778	3,913
1994	7	49	388	12	102	426	27	319	1,619	68	865	4,364
1995	3	48	387	13	111	420	36	388	1,763	74	1,027	4,602
Cumbria												
1981-85	5	22	62	13	127	355	16	195	605	55	675	2,043
1994	3	18	65	12	91	330	18	155	630	43	431	1,825
1995	3	20	85	14	80	343	17	150	573	50	442	1,899
Greater Manchester												
1981-85	10	59	337	6	50	214	90	971	4,966	178	2,149	11,127
1994	11	53	564	5	28	253	45	581	5,522	107	1,338	12,373
1995	10	50	546	4	17	219	54	538	5,315	110	1,226	11,917
Lancashire												
1981-85	8	40	147	17	113	377	60	554	2,161	135	1,478	5,803
1994	7	63	258	12	107	443	39	517	2,348	101	1,482	6,409
1995	5	48	220	7	86	391	42	522	2,178	94	1,451	6,155
Merseyside												
1981-85	3	14	67	7	59	260	50	406	2,059	107	1,099	5,756
1994	2	16	158	6	43	397	38	314	2,677	74	840	6,974
1995	3	15	148	6	34	347	24	297	2,383	59	733	6,447
Yorkshire and Humberside Region												
1981-85	14	78	306	65	541	1,498	196	2,053	6,932	463	5,714	20,018
1994	10	56	559	33	339	1,378	136	1,258	7,055	294	3,627	20,121
1995	14	90	560	41	303	1,344	119	1,318	6,943	313	3,709	19,954
Humberside												
1981-85	2	10	33	8	72	243	28	308	1,201	73	996	3,894
1994	2	10	57	3	53	201	23	199	972	53	748	3,718
1995	0	6	28	7	34	187	21	224	1,020	64	758	3,685
North Yorkshire												
1981-85	0	3	8	24	239	467	29	474	1,048	82	1,423	3,128
1994	0	1	5	16	180	521	33	310	1,100	73	912	3,156
1995	1	2	5	20	163	510	29	300	1,097	77	872	3,194

1 This county contains no motorways.

14 Accidents: by road class, severity, Government Office Region and county: 1981-85 average, 1994, 1995

Number

	Motorways			Trunk A roads			Principal A roads			All roads		
	Fatal	Fatal or serious	All severities	Fatal	Fatal or serious	All severities	Fatal	Fatal or serious	All severities	Fatal	Fatal or serious	All severities
South Yorkshire												
1981-85	4	26	110	10	75	250	42	420	1,654	103	1,123	4,631
1994	4	22	177	4	22	143	28	264	1,786	57	617	4,629
1995	5	39	184	2	25	137	21	234	1,595	53	644	4,374
West Yorkshire												
1981-85	7	39	155	23	155	538	96	851	3,030	205	2,172	8,365
1994	4	23	320	10	84	513	52	485	3,197	111	1,350	8,618
1995	8	43	343	12	81	510	48	560	3,231	119	1,435	8,701
East Midlands Region												
1981-85	15	129	390	97	792	2,350	158	1,770	5,721	443	5,334	17,379
1994	4	72	428	65	461	2,026	113	1,114	5,369	308	3,231	16,091
1995	9	80	393	69	486	1,967	123	1,188	5,397	340	3,466	15,902
Derbyshire												
1981-85	2	18	69	20	159	545	34	339	1,130	97	1,057	3,743
1994	1	14	119	12	87	521	21	149	1,107	53	481	3,619
1995	2	13	117	5	102	522	20	218	1,083	52	728	3,554
Leicestershire												
1981-85	6	24	93	16	115	360	32	330	1,198	93	1,042	3,702
1994	1	13	146	10	43	288	23	194	1,190	71	515	3,546
1995	4	30	149	16	53	286	14	154	1,157	69	511	3,515
Lincolnshire[1]												
1981-85	0	0	0	20	160	454	29	294	932	76	852	2,683
1994	0	0	0	9	89	316	34	215	852	73	597	2,441
1995	0	0	0	13	71	299	36	226	953	76	574	2,531
Northamptonshire												
1981-85	6	75	190	18	182	434	22	381	1,011	69	1,025	2,673
1994	2	38	117	11	99	317	9	222	812	34	614	2,196
1995	3	33	85	10	110	303	14	245	849	42	638	2,104
Nottinghamshire												
1981-85	1	11	38	22	175	557	41	426	1,450	108	1,359	4,577
1994	0	7	46	23	143	584	26	334	1,408	77	1,024	4,289
1995	0	4	42	25	150	557	39	345	1,355	101	1,015	4,198
Eastern Region												
1981-85	15	116	440	101	840	2,481	172	2,170	7,213	480	6,885	22,569
1994	19	119	806	63	524	2,262	121	1,362	6,971	341	4,385	21,535
1995	19	138	974	95	573	2,383	103	1,288	6,678	340	4,248	21,074
Bedfordshire												
1981-85	4	29	109	10	94	345	17	160	622	50	600	2,444
1994	2	10	93	6	57	278	13	104	531	37	362	2,018
1995	3	17	117	18	63	310	6	88	528	42	334	1,951
Cambridgeshire												
1981-85	1	5	19	23	158	462	25	303	1,009	75	908	2,979
1994	0	2	16	18	115	487	23	224	1,092	66	699	3,221
1995	0	1	12	28	135	557	21	186	1,015	72	615	3,197
Essex												
1981-85	3	29	109	11	97	321	53	675	2,398	125	2,032	6,976
1994	6	49	304	9	97	478	26	355	2,241	85	1,287	6,934
1995	9	45	291	10	89	450	27	382	2,187	85	1,285	6,769
Hertfordshire												
1981-85	7	53	203	16	121	404	30	393	1,469	84	1,177	4,316
1994	11	58	393	6	73	395	19	249	1,330	51	779	4,249
1995	7	75	554	5	88	390	19	251	1,395	42	870	4,493
Norfolk[1]												
1981-85	0	0	0	21	190	461	27	360	910	82	1,207	3,110
1994	0	0	0	14	137	400	25	272	982	59	828	3,018
1995	0	0	0	22	129	356	24	262	922	67	753	2,652

1 This county contains no motorways.

14 Accidents: by road class, severity, Government Office Region and county: 1981-85 average, 1994, 1995

	Motorways			Trunk A roads			Principal A roads			All roads		
	Fatal	Fatal or serious	All severities	Fatal	Fatal or serious	All severities	Fatal	Fatal or serious	All severities	Fatal	Fatal or serious	All severities
Suffolk[1]												
1981-85	0	0	0	20	179	488	19	280	805	64	960	2,744
1994	0	0	0	10	45	224	15	158	795	43	430	2,095
1995	0	0	0	12	69	320	6	119	631	32	391	2,012
South East Region												
1981-85	34	243	771	112	836	2,563	308	3,818	13,093	740	10,169	34,809
1994	20	212	1,644	61	420	2,170	211	2,090	12,176	444	5,417	32,549
1995	26	249	1,740	56	396	2,115	189	2,041	11,948	431	5,295	32,037
Berkshire												
1981-85	10	69	215	7	61	195	24	321	1,167	71	942	3,263
1994	5	26	230	0	12	123	25	144	1,073	47	337	2,924
1995	3	31	292	2	7	122	10	104	1,074	32	293	3,007
Buckinghamshire												
1981-85	5	38	120	3	36	110	27	318	1,001	63	843	2,617
1994	3	21	214	5	25	136	21	114	890	38	330	2,725
1995	2	26	204	2	16	144	18	115	817	39	322	2,561
East Sussex[1]												
1981-85	0	0	0	10	78	232	31	347	1,163	66	838	2,997
1994	0	0	0	12	59	258	13	222	1,230	38	549	3,054
1995	0	0	0	2	62	248	19	203	1,122	37	510	2,916
Hampshire												
1981-85	4	36	109	21	160	437	50	792	2,416	140	2,320	7,227
1994	6	52	285	8	62	309	34	425	2,273	74	1,205	6,761
1995	7	61	358	10	82	329	26	416	2,233	68	1,160	6,834
Isle of Wight[1]												
1981-85	0	0	0	0	0	0	4	70	214	8	155	495
1994	0	0	0	0	0	0	3	44	203	5	94	471
1995	0	0	0	0	0	0	4	43	205	6	96	476
Kent												
1981-85	7	49	162	21	175	539	63	779	2,543	142	2,053	6,819
1994	1	35	219	9	114	566	39	444	2,378	80	1,230	6,161
1995	6	56	236	18	103	470	34	481	2,403	81	1,219	5,814
Oxfordshire												
1981-85	1	6	12	24	164	521	26	279	801	71	871	2,531
1994	3	18	129	9	44	262	24	139	815	46	336	2,202
1995	5	21	107	10	39	287	23	129	806	57	322	2,230
Surrey												
1981-85	7	43	144	10	62	224	52	613	2,618	109	1,391	5,870
1994	2	59	546	8	41	242	33	352	2,254	67	819	5,497
1995	2	50	516	6	39	256	40	329	2,232	72	843	5,444
West Sussex												
1981-85	0	2	9	16	102	306	31	299	1,170	70	757	2,990
1994	0	1	21	10	63	274	19	206	1,060	49	517	2,754
1995	1	4	27	6	48	259	15	221	1,056	39	530	2,755
London Region												
1981-85	6	35	266	56	413	2,489	301	4,269	25,584	521	7,588	45,274
1994	4	75	527	42	637	4,406	137	2,857	19,368	264	5,659	38,527
1995	7	64	438	25	640	4,349	102	2,962	18,945	203	5,922	37,978
Inner London												
1981-85[2]	..	..	..	..	..	..	..	..	..	212	3,383	20,946
1994	0	12	75	22	272	1,701	70	1,568	10,198	117	2,756	17,693
1995	2	7	61	10	249	1,671	51	1,550	10,105	87	2,686	17,453
Outer London												
1981-85[2]	..	..	..	..	..	..	..	..	..	309	4,204	24,327
1994	4	63	452	20	365	2,705	67	1,289	9,170	147	2,903	20,834
1995	5	57	377	15	391	2,678	51	1,412	8,840	116	3,236	20,525

1 This county contains no motorways.
2 Trunk road data not available for these years.

14 Accidents: by road class, severity, Government Office Region and county: 1981-85 average, 1994, 1995

Number

	Motorways			Trunk A roads			Principal A roads			All roads		
	Fatal	Fatal or serious	All severities	Fatal	Fatal or serious	All severities	Fatal	Fatal or serious	All severities	Fatal	Fatal or serious	All severities
South West Region												
1981-85	17	127	344	62	585	1,586	198	2,475	7,389	440	6,697	19,847
1994	14	79	427	52	251	1,249	128	1,090	6,169	294	3,017	17,150
1995	19	78	478	31	212	1,232	147	1,059	6,196	319	2,843	17,272
Avon												
1981-85	8	50	124	3	29	61	41	450	1,415	86	1,149	3,596
1994	5	23	183	3	8	42	15	122	926	39	401	2,711
1995	8	32	210	3	7	56	30	168	1,091	61	459	3,144
Cornwall[1]												
1981-85	0	0	0	10	92	249	14	236	667	39	696	1,984
1994	0	0	0	6	47	225	13	141	725	27	386	2,002
1995	0	0	0	4	31	200	18	120	645	31	297	1,816
Devon												
1981-85	2	10	27	13	131	345	35	570	1,563	82	1,568	4,354
1994	0	10	43	11	55	289	12	218	1,166	40	682	3,933
1995	2	7	41	4	45	303	10	184	1,145	39	602	3,908
Dorset[1]												
1981-85	0	0	0	4	45	148	23	311	1,112	48	803	2,779
1994	0	0	0	3	26	153	19	159	1,024	42	394	2,497
1995	0	0	0	5	31	142	20	148	1,045	43	382	2,463
Gloucestershire												
1981-85	1	21	54	13	145	369	24	282	705	59	967	2,479
1994	3	9	53	15	49	244	20	124	725	50	341	1,990
1995	1	7	63	4	43	251	22	102	639	40	304	1,923
Somerset												
1981-85	3	17	43	6	48	117	29	295	789	57	666	1,783
1994	3	13	60	4	15	57	20	139	711	39	339	1,697
1995	4	7	52	3	10	58	24	164	748	51	339	1,737
Wiltshire												
1981-85	4	28	96	12	94	297	32	331	1,138	68	847	2,871
1994	3	24	88	10	51	239	29	187	892	57	474	2,320
1995	4	25	112	8	45	222	23	173	883	54	460	2,281
West Midlands Region												
1981-85	19	137	476	80	639	1,827	191	2,263	7,415	484	6,527	21,030
1994	15	168	789	63	391	1,623	160	1,584	7,543	348	4,420	20,571
1995	17	145	777	40	342	1,552	110	1,408	7,211	265	4,000	20,030
Hereford and Worcester												
1981-85	4	29	104	10	83	245	31	329	1,060	71	859	2,762
1994	2	32	103	8	87	295	30	268	932	58	730	2,599
1995	1	34	111	9	76	286	21	260	981	40	688	2,641
Shropshire												
1981-85	0	2	4	14	147	363	17	170	473	51	653	1,611
1994	0	3	10	14	76	216	13	145	451	38	471	1,514
1995	2	3	18	7	66	220	8	126	435	27	425	1,534
Staffordshire												
1981-85	8	36	146	25	163	602	36	405	1,577	105	1,209	4,813
1994	8	39	232	22	98	622	46	238	1,803	92	668	4,928
1995	6	14	203	9	73	554	28	197	1,713	69	536	4,708
Warwickshire												
1981-85	4	29	68	19	148	336	23	220	553	77	850	2,078
1994	2	49	206	14	77	256	13	149	600	48	621	2,321
1995	4	58	209	14	70	258	8	131	555	41	543	2,221
West Midlands												
1981-85	4	41	154	12	98	280	84	1,140	3,752	180	2,956	9,767
1994	3	45	238	5	53	234	58	784	3,757	112	1,930	9,209
1995	4	36	236	1	57	234	45	694	3,527	88	1,808	8,926

1 This county contains no motorways.

14 Accidents: by road class, severity, Government Office Region and county: 1981-85 average, 1994, 1995

Number

	Motorways			Trunk A roads			Principal A roads			All roads		
	Fatal	Fatal or serious	All severities	Fatal	Fatal or serious	All severities	Fatal	Fatal or serious	All severities	Fatal	Fatal or serious	All severities
England												
1981-85	156	1,059	3,860	654	5,220	16,880	1,859	22,035	87,572	4,333	57,347	218,137
1994	118	993	6,716	439	3,500	17,539	1,223	13,723	80,192	2,813	36,194	206,788
1995	141	1,041	6,851	410	3,369	17,279	1,126	13,622	78,317	2,733	35,671	203,576
Wales												
1981-85	5	38	124	62	620	1,746	86	984	3,427	233	3,082	10,583
1994	6	26	179	48	329	1,487	73	570	3,201	194	1,776	10,536
1995	4	28	209	49	323	1,382	75	502	2,956	193	1,677	10,275
Scotland												
1981-85	16	110	265	138	1,010	2,433	228	2,751	7,438	581	7,412	20,471
1994	11	99	330	86	631	1,894	121	1,520	5,568	319	4,642	16,777
1995	9	84	332	94	619	1,857	133	1,521	5,540	360	4,429	16,525
Great Britain												
1981-85	177	1,207	4,249	854	6,850	21,058	2,173	25,769	98,436	5,147	67,842	249,192
1994	135	1,118	7,225	573	4,460	20,920	1,417	15,813	88,961	3,326	42,612	234,101
1995	154	1,153	7,392	553	4,311	20,518	1,334	15,645	86,813	3,286	41,777	230,376

15 Accidents and casualties by severity: vehicles involved by vehicle type: road length: all by selected individual motorways[1]: 1995

Number

	Accidents			Casualties			Vehicles involved				Kilo-metres open at December 1995[3]
	Fatal	Serious	All severities	Fatal	Serious	All severities	Two-wheel motor vehicles	Cars and LGV	HGV	All vehicles[2]	
England											
M1 / M10	20	144	980	23	194	1,658	43	1,965	334	2,372	319
M45	0	1	3	0	1	7	1	2	1	4	13
M2	0	12	59	0	12	87	5	94	19	120	43
M3	1	37	229	1	43	353	23	410	32	468	90
M4	11	73	603	23	110	936	46	1,086	108	1,269	187
M5	11	56	373	11	78	591	17	701	107	833	262
M6	24	129	940	26	191	1,659	31	1,681	395	2,150	383
M11	3	18	143	3	23	209	11	225	38	278	85
M18	2	7	50	3	10	85	2	84	19	108	46
M20	4	23	98	4	34	186	1	154	30	185	86
M23	1	11	85	1	14	146	6	161	12	182	27
M25	16	109	1,028	17	139	1,623	52	2,036	302	2,420	185
M26	0	4	12	0	4	24	1	17	3	21	16
M27 / M271 / M275	6	27	206	6	38	299	17	443	25	490	60
M40	6	45	273	7	60	454	9	487	64	566	147
M42	1	27	112	1	34	174	5	203	28	239	72
M50	0	4	11	0	4	14	0	9	7	16	35
M53	0	8	76	0	8	120	2	137	8	149	33
M54	2	2	29	2	2	39	2	47	10	61	36
M55	0	4	19	0	7	40	0	29	5	34	19
M56	1	12	108	1	12	171	2	182	31	220	58
M57	2	1	26	2	2	50	0	50	2	52	17
M58	0	1	24	0	1	30	2	32	6	40	19
M61	2	11	72	2	17	116	3	128	19	151	40
M62	11	48	483	15	61	753	19	870	186	1,081	174
M63	1	7	132	1	8	192	1	259	30	294	26
M65	0	7	30	0	8	45	0	55	4	61	22
M66	0	7	39	0	7	53	2	84	5	93	19
M69	0	4	27	0	5	36	2	37	5	44	28
M180 / M181	1	4	19	1	4	20	0	16	9	26	45
Other motorways	3	6	112	3	6	148	10	201	14	228	36
Motorways	129	849	6,401	153	1,137	10,318	315	11,885	1,858	14,255	2,625
A(M) roads	12	51	450	13	63	673	29	821	78	937	201
Total (inc A(M) roads)	141	900	6,851	166	1,200	10,991	344	12,706	1,936	15,192	2,826
Wales											
Motorways	4	24	209	4	34	323	6	404	57	475	..
A(M) roads	0	0	0	0	0	0	0	0	0	0	..
Total (inc A(M) roads)	4	24	209	4	34	323	6	404	57	475	126
Scotland											
Motorways	9	75	330	10	99	535	12	554	73	648	..
A(M) roads	0	0	2	0	0	2	0	2	0	3	..
Total (inc A(M) roads)	9	75	332	10	99	537	12	556	73	651	316
Great Britain											
Motorways	142	948	6,940	167	1,270	11,176	333	12,843	1,988	15,378	..
A(M) roads	12	51	452	13	63	675	29	823	78	940	..
Total (inc A(M) roads)	154	999	7,392	180	1,333	11,851	362	13,666	2,066	16,318	3,268

1 Casualty and accident data by road class are not available for Northern Ireland.
2 Includes pedal cycles, buses and coaches and other vehicles.
3 Excluding slip roads. Data for England from 1994 onwards supplied by DOT Statistics Directorate. Data for Wales from Welsh Office and Scotland from Scottish Office.

16 Distribution of accidents by road class and Government Office Region[1]: 1994, 1995

percentage (row sums = 100)

	Motorways		Trunk roads		Principal roads		Other roads	
	1994	1995	1994	1995	1994	1995	1994	1995
North East	1.2	1.3	6.9	7.4	33.1	33.5	58.7	57.8
North West	5.1	5.0	5.8	5.6	40.5	40.0	48.6	49.4
Merseyside	2.3	2.3	5.7	5.4	38.4	37.0	53.7	55.4
North West/Merseyside	4.5	4.5	5.8	5.5	40.1	39.4	49.7	50.6
Yorkshire/Humberside	2.8	2.8	6.8	6.7	35.1	34.8	55.3	55.7
East Midlands	2.7	2.5	12.6	12.4	33.4	33.9	51.4	51.2
West Midlands	3.8	3.9	7.9	7.7	36.7	36.0	51.6	52.4
Eastern	3.7	4.6	10.5	11.3	32.4	31.7	53.4	52.4
South East	5.1	5.4	6.7	6.6	37.4	37.3	50.9	50.7
London	1.4	1.2	11.4	11.5	50.3	49.9	36.9	37.5
South West	2.5	2.8	7.3	7.1	36.0	35.9	54.3	54.2
England	3.2	3.4	8.5	8.5	38.8	38.5	49.5	49.7
Wales	1.7	2.0	14.1	13.5	30.4	28.8	53.8	55.7
Scotland	2.0	2.0	11.3	11.2	33.2	33.5	53.6	53.2
Great Britain	3.1	3.2	8.9	8.9	38.0	37.7	50.0	50.2

1 Accident data by road class are not available for Northern Ireland.

17 Motor vehicles, population, area and road length (motorways and built-up and non built-up roads: by trunk and principal): by Government Office Region: 1995

Thousands/ number

	Motor vehicles currently licensed[1] (thousands)	Population[2] mid year (home) (thousands)	Area in hectares (thousands)	Road length (kilometres)				
				Motorways[3 4]	Built-up[4]		Non built-up[4]	
					Trunk	Principal	Trunk	Principal
North East	888	2,610	859	55	12	505	423	886
North West	2,387	5,468	1,351	518	113	1,455	702	1,485
Merseyside	467	1,434	66	61	24	310	45	56
North West/Merseyside	2,853	6,902	1,417	579	137	1,765	748	1,540
Yorkshire/Humberside	2,006	5,026	1,541	298	93	1,192	651	1,486
East Midlands	1,764	4,103	1,563	190	139	781	1,107	1,956
West Midlands	2,590	5,295	1,300	375	100	1,083	749	1,676
Eastern	2,704	5,224	1,912	236	71	999	1,172	1,886
South East	3,822	7,786	1,910	658	78	1,765	829	2,750
London	2,684	6,967	158	62	203	1,358	123	44
South West	2,417	4,796	2,383	295	53	1,139	994	2,923
England	21,730	48,708	13,042	2,748	885	10,586	6,796	15,147
Wales	1,175	2,913	2,077	126	198	867	1,379	1,801
Scotland	1,910	5,132	7,717	316	215	1,307	2,636	6,258
Great Britain	24,815	56,753	22,836	3,189	1,297	12,760	10,811	23,206
Northern Ireland	612	1,642	1,416	112	500[5]		1,725[5]	
United Kingdom	25,427	58,395	24,252	3,301	1,297	12,760	10,811	23,206

1 Includes all vehicles licensed to use public roads. From 1992, estimates of licensed stock are taken from the Department of Transport's Statistics Directorate Information Database.
2 Final 1994 population estimates.
3 Data for Wales from Welsh Office and Scotland from Scottish Office.
4 As at April 1995. Road length figures taken from DOT Transport Statistics Report "Road Lengths in Great Britain 1995".
5 Trunk and Principal road length data are not available for Northern Ireland, data are for all A roads.

18 Motor traffic distribution between Government Office Regions[1]: by motorway and built-up and non built-up trunk and principal roads: 1993-1995 average

Percentage[2]

	Motorways	Built-up A		Non built-up A		All major roads
		Trunk	Principal	Trunk	Principal	
North East	1	1	3	5	5	3
North West	16	6	12	6	8	11
Merseyside	1	2	3	1	0	1
North West/Merseyside	17	9	15	7	8	12
Yorkshire/Humberside	8	7	9	8	7	8
East Midlands	6	11	5	11	9	8
West Midlands	13	8	10	7	8	9
Eastern	10	6	7	17	13	11
South East	25	6	14	13	21	18
London	3	33	16	4	1	7
South West	8	3	8	9	13	9
England	92	83	88	80	84	86
Wales	3	8	4	7	5	5
Scotland	5	9	8	13	11	9
Great Britain	100	100	100	100	100	100

1 Traffic data by road class are not available for Northern Ireland.
2 Figures have been rounded to the nearest whole number.

19 Motor traffic distribution between motorways, built-up and non built-up trunk and principal roads: by Government Office Region[1]: 1993-1995 average

Percentage[2]

	Motorways	Built-up A		Non built-up A		All major roads
		Trunk	Principal	Trunk	Principal	
North East	9	1	26	31	33	100
North West	38	2	31	13	16	100
Merseyside	24	7	50	12	7	100
North West/Merseyside	37	3	33	13	15	100
Yorkshire/Humberside	24	3	30	22	20	100
East Midlands	20	5	18	31	26	100
West Midlands	35	3	27	16	18	100
Eastern	22	2	17	33	26	100
South East	35	1	21	17	26	100
London	10	16	57	14	2	100
South West	23	1	22	22	32	100
England	27	3	27	21	22	100
Wales	15	6	23	32	24	100
Scotland	15	4	23	32	26	100
Great Britain	25	4	26	23	23	100

1 Traffic data by road class are not available for Northern Ireland.
2 Figures have been rounded to the nearest whole number.

ANNEX A

HIGHWAYS AGENCY
TABLES

A1: Casualties: by Highways Agency Region and severity: 1981-85 average, 1988-1995; rate per 100,000 population, 1995

Number/rate

	1981-85 Average	1988	1989	1990	1991	1992	1993	1994	1995	Rate per 100,000 Population[1]
Northern										
Killed	1,429	1,298	1,378	1,331	1,241	1,158	1,072	942	977	6
Killed or Seriously Injured	17,736	15,074	15,231	15,218	13,393	13,068	12,058	12,408	12,481	81
All Casualties	78,239	82,151	88,491	90,535	84,747	86,516	85,425	89,134	87,454	565
Midlands										
Killed	1,356	1,222	1,371	1,363	1,136	1,089	970	1,008	953	8
Killed or Seriously Injured	19,751	16,116	16,343	15,956	13,293	12,666	11,634	12,321	11,375	93
All Casualties	67,620	69,031	73,506	73,667	66,491	65,941	64,685	65,696	64,222	525
Southern										
Killed	1,374	1,317	1,378	1,320	1,109	986	900	857	855	6
Killed or Seriously Injured	21,669	17,547	16,895	15,724	12,850	12,337	11,685	11,503	11,338	81
All Casualties	80,363	80,691	83,176	81,282	73,081	72,958	73,355	76,984	76,876	548
London										
Killed	539	446	460	409	368	316	286	270	210	3
Killed or Seriously Injured	8,229	9,478	9,344	8,923	7,868	7,226	6,413	6,171	6,482	93
All Casualties	54,154	50,114	52,779	51,992	46,523	46,344	45,822	45,687	44,821	643

1 Based on final 1994 population estimates.

A2 Number of casualties: by Highways Agency Region and road user type: 1981-85 average, 1995

Number of casualties

	Children (0-15)	Adults (16-59)	Elderly (60+)	All[1] casualties	Pedest-rians	Pedal cyclists	Motor cyclists	Car occupants	Other[2] road users
Northern									
1981-85	14,773	54,863	8,315	78,239	18,074	6,905	15,060	32,194	6,006
1995	13,940	64,481	8,816	87,454	14,090	6,438	4,604	55,762	6,560
Midlands									
1981-85	10,507	50,615	6,436	67,620	10,843	6,728	14,715	31,120	4,213
1995	9,006	47,612	6,434	64,222	8,305	5,422	4,865	41,588	4,042
Southern									
1981-85	10,746	61,029	8,261	80,363	10,516	7,555	19,446	38,710	4,135
1995	9,442	58,022	7,951	76,876	8,587	6,474	6,791	50,777	4,247
London									
1981-85	7,106	37,830	5,854	54,154	13,081	4,739	9,957	21,776	4,601
1995	5,209	32,308	3,945	44,821	9,371	4,512	5,437	22,055	3,446

1 Includes age not reported.
2 Includes road user type not known.

A3 Total casualty rates[1]: by Highways Agency Region and road user type: 1995

Rate per 100,000 population

	Children (0-15)	Adults (16-59)	Elderly (60+)	All[2] casualties	Pedest-rians	Pedal cyclists	Motor cyclists	Car occupants	Other[3] road users
Northern	8,998	41,622	5,691	56,451	9,095	4,156	2,972	35,994	4,234
Midlands	7,363	38,923	5,260	52,502	6,789	4,433	3,977	33,999	3,304
Southern	6,736	41,395	5,673	54,847	6,126	4,619	4,845	36,227	3,030
London	7,477	46,374	5,663	64,335	13,451	6,476	7,804	31,657	4,946

1 Based on final 1994 population estimates.
2 Includes age not reported.
3 Includes road user type not known.

A4 Casualty indicators: by Highways Agency Region and road user type: 1995

								Percentage of all casualties
	Percentage of all casualties who are:							
	Children[1] (0-15)	Adults[1] (16-59)	Elderly[1] (60+)	Pedest- rians	Pedal cyclists	Motor cyclists	Car occupants	Other[2] road users
Northern	16.0	73.9	10.1	16.1	7.4	5.3	63.8	7.5
Midlands	14.3	75.5	10.2	12.9	8.4	7.6	64.8	6.3
Southern	12.5	76.9	10.5	11.2	8.4	8.8	66.1	5.5
London	12.6	77.9	9.5	20.9	10.1	12.1	49.2	7.7

1 Percentage of casualties of known age.
2 Includes road user type not known.

A5: Casualty changes: by Highways Agency Region and severity: 1981-85 average, 1995

						Number of casualties
	Fatal and serious casualties			Total casualties		
	1981-85 average	1995	Percentage change	1981-85 average	1995	Percentage change
Northern	17,736	12,481	-29.6	78,239	87,454	11.8
Midlands	19,751	11,375	-42.4	67,620	64,222	-5.0
Southern	21,669	11,338	-47.7	80,363	76,876	-4.3
London	8,229	6,482	-21.2	54,154	44,821	-17.2

A6: Number of casualties: by road class, Highways Agency Region and severity: 1995

											Number of casualties
		Built-Up					Non Built-Up				
	Motorways	Trunk	Principal	Other	Total		Trunk	Principal	Other	Total	All Roads[1]
Northern											
Killed	54	15	222	275	512		104	191	116	411	977
Killed or Seriously Injured	380	235	3,004	4,920	8,159		892	1,639	1,411	3,942	12,481
All Casualties	3,490	2,098	25,462	38,001	65,561		4,556	7,594	6,253	18,403	87,454
Midlands											
Killed	36	18	135	155	308		207	217	185	609	953
Killed or Seriously Injured	343	278	2,115	3,563	5,956		1,335	1,850	1,891	5,076	11,375
All Casualties	2,208	1,803	14,380	23,096	39,279		6,184	8,237	8,313	22,734	64,222
Southern											
Killed	71	7	118	148	273		88	246	174	508	855
Killed or Seriously Injured	591	151	1,991	3,583	5,725		717	2,157	2,145	5,019	11,338
All Casualties	4,856	1,160	16,093	27,018	44,271		4,406	11,754	11,573	27,733	76,876
London											
Killed	5	21	102	74	197		4	4	0	8	210
Killed or Seriously Injured	52	595	3,191	2,424	6,210		150	41	29	220	6,482
All Casualties	437	4,523	22,014	16,555	43,092		934	191	166	1,291	44,821

1 Includes speed limit not reported.

A7: Casualty rates per 100 million vehicle kilometres: by road class, Highways Agency Region and severity: 1993-1995 average

Rate per 100 million vehicle kilometres

	Motorways	A Roads Built-Up Trunk	A Roads Built-Up Principle	A Roads Non Built-Up Trunk	A Roads Non Built-Up Principle	All A Roads	All major roads[1]
Northern							
Killed	0.3	1.1	1.2	0.8	1.5	1.2	0.9
Killed or Seriously Injured	2.0	12.6	15.1	7.1	11.9	12.0	9.2
All Casualties	18.6	109.6	128.2	35.9	58.6	83.6	65.3
Midlands							
Killed	0.3	1.0	1.1	1.1	1.6	1.3	1.0
Killed or Seriously Injured	2.4	13.1	16.6	7.7	13.1	12.1	9.7
All Casualties	14.9	94.7	109.9	35.1	57.0	65.1	52.8
Southern							
Killed	0.2	1.2	0.8	0.7	1.1	0.9	0.7
Killed or Seriously Injured	2.2	16.4	12.2	5.2	9.6	9.3	7.1
All Casualties	17.5	124.9	94.1	29.7	52.1	60.1	46.6
London							
Killed	0.2	1.0	1.2	0.3	0.8	1.0	0.9
Killed or Seriously Injured	3.3	19.0	29.1	5.8	11.1	23.2	21.2
All Casualties	25.6	143.7	207.6	36.8	69.8	166.2	151.7

1 Includes road class and type not reported.

A8: Accident rates per 100 million vehicle kilometres: by road class, Highways Agency Region and severity: 1993-1995 average

Rate per 100 million vehicle kilometres

	Motorways	A Roads Built-Up Trunk	A Roads Built-Up Principle	A Roads Non Built-Up Trunk	A Roads Non Built-Up Principle	All A Roads	All Major Roads[1]
Northern							
Killed	0.3	1.0	1.1	0.7	1.3	1.1	0.8
Killed or Seriously Injured	1.5	11.1	13.5	5.0	8.8	9.8	7.5
All Casualties	11.4	78.4	93.4	21.1	35.7	57.6	44.6
Midlands							
Killed	0.2	0.9	1.0	1.0	1.4	1.1	0.9
Killed or Seriously Injured	1.7	11.3	14.6	5.6	9.7	9.6	7.7
All Casualties	9.0	70.2	83.9	21.2	36.1	45.2	36.3
Southern							
Killed	0.2	1.2	0.8	0.6	1.0	0.8	0.6
Killed or Seriously Injured	1.7	13.9	11.1	4.0	7.4	7.7	5.8
All Casualties	10.8	92.0	73.8	18.8	34.0	43.1	32.8
London							
Killed	0.2	0.9	1.2	0.3	0.7	1.0	0.9
Killed or Seriously Injured	2.6	16.5	26.8	4.7	9.1	21.1	19.2
All Casualties	19.0	116.2	176.8	26.8	52.9	139.6	127.1

1 Includes road class and type not reported.

A9: Accidents and accident indices[1]: by month, severity and Highways Agency Region: 1995

Index/number

	Jan	Feb	Mar	Apr	May	Jun	Jul	Aug	Sep	Oct	Nov	Dec	All Accidents
Northern													
Fatal or Serious	93.1	93.0	96.2	93.3	93.1	98.2	99.6	103.1	110.5	102.8	113.4	103.5	10,625
All severities	96.0	95.6	101.2	87.0	95.7	94.0	97.5	99.3	109.3	102.8	113.3	108.0	62,837
Midlands													
Fatal or Serious	94.9	93.3	101.7	92.5	92.1	106.0	91.9	101.6	107.4	106.3	115.9	96.4	9,457
All severities	99.0	95.7	97.4	86.1	94.1	99.4	96.7	98.1	111.6	104.2	116.3	101.6	46,343
Southern													
Fatal or Serious	90.6	95.9	97.8	94.2	96.6	100.9	105.6	101.0	109.6	102.2	111.2	94.4	9,690
All severities	93.5	98.1	97.5	86.0	95.0	99.5	101.5	99.7	109.4	102.5	117.1	100.3	56,539
London													
Fatal or Serious	85.0	78.2	82.2	103.1	102.2	106.8	106.0	95.0	103.5	114.6	113.0	109.0	5,899
All severities	95.4	108.4	106.5	89.4	99.2	101.3	97.5	96.4	111.5	95.4	108.2	91.8	37,857

1 The base (= 100) is the average number of accidents per day for the region.

A10: Accidents on motorways: by carriageway type, junction, number of lanes, Highways Agency Region and severity: 1995

Number of accidents

	Junction			Non-junction		
	Number of lanes		Circular section of roundabouts	Number of lanes		Total[1]
	2	3+		2	3+	
Northern						
Fatal or Serious	15	17	7	39	194	300
All severities	145	120	173	222	1,255	2,168
Midlands						
Fatal or Serious	3	23	2	16	207	258
All severities	23	105	49	60	1,032	1,352
Southern						
Fatal or Serious	14	30	4	49	307	442
All severities	101	228	86	288	2,026	3,014
London						
Fatal or Serious	7	11	0	6	16	41
All severities	54	64	9	60	119	317

1 Includes unknown carriageway type and slip roads.

A11: Accidents on trunk A roads: by carriageway type, junction, number of lanes, Highways Agency Region and severity: 1995

Number of accidents

	Dual carriageway					Single carriageway							Circular Section of round-about	All Trunk A Roads[5]
	Junction[4]		Non-junction			Junction[4]			Non-junction					
	Number of lanes[1]		Number of lanes[1]			Number of lanes[2]			Number of lanes[2]					
	2	3+	2	3+	All	2[3]	3	4+	2[3]	3	4+	All		
Northern														
Fatal or Serious	85	28	144	15	272	202	18	19	257	9	7	512	36	822
All Severities	565	159	673	96	1,493	1,037	92	124	879	30	33	2,195	485	4,203
Midlands														
Fatal or Serious	163	9	235	11	418	307	28	18	343	4	9	709	74	1,204
All Severities	608	54	962	44	1,668	1,386	91	65	1,092	23	34	2,691	702	5,078
Southern														
Fatal or Serious	95	26	154	37	312	135	6	2	176	14	2	335	47	703
All Severities	406	118	811	210	1,545	685	53	9	703	45	14	1,509	554	3,649
London														
Fatal or Serious	79	119	64	65	327	163	10	31	66	6	8	284	27	640
All Severities	607	718	351	441	2,117	1,122	56	249	357	25	69	1,878	311	4,349

1 Number of lanes in each direction.
2 Number of lanes in both directions.
3 Includes one way streets.
4 Does not include accidents at roundabouts.
5 Includes unknown carriageway type and single track roads.

A12: Accidents on principal A roads: by carriageway type, junction, number of lanes, Highways Agency Region and severity: 1995

Number of accidents

	Dual carriageway					Single carriageway							Circular Section of round-about	All Trunk A Roads[5]
	Junction[4]		Non-junction			Junction[4]			Non-junction					
	Number of lanes[1]		Number of lanes[1]			Number of lanes[2]			Number of lanes[2]					
	2	3+	2	3+	All	2[3]	3	4+	2[3]	3	4+	All		
Northern														
Fatal or Serious	284	113	206	44	647	1,522	120	119	1,216	38	35	3,050	167	3,894
All Severities	2,346	875	1,033	252	4,506	9,694	627	940	4,860	143	198	16,462	1,669	23,025
Midlands														
Fatal or Serious	222	50	188	25	485	1,230	58	124	1,139	20	49	2,620	151	3,264
All Severities	1,375	342	769	69	2,555	6,636	312	585	4,230	87	179	12,029	1,414	16,066
Southern														
Fatal or Serious	224	39	224	27	514	1,275	55	38	1,272	39	17	2,696	246	3,502
All Severities	1,404	268	1,155	123	2,950	8,010	355	247	5,551	150	87	14,400	2,576	20,281
London														
Fatal or Serious	184	73	92	27	376	1,584	60	288	463	17	55	2,467	87	2,962
All Severities	1,290	363	438	117	2,208	10,308	323	1,666	3,005	77	394	15,773	768	18,945

1 Number of lanes in each direction.
2 Number of lanes in both directions.
3 Includes one way streets.
4 Does not include accidents at roundabouts.
5 Includes unknown carriageway type and single track roads.

A13: Accidents: by road class, severity, Highways Agency Region: 1981-85 average, 1994, 1995

Number of accidents

	Motorways			Trunk A roads			Principal A roads			All roads		
	Fatal	Fatal or serious	All severities	Fatal	Fatal or serious	All severities	Fatal	Fatal or serious	All severities	Fatal	Fatal or serious	All severities
Northern												
1981-85	53	291	1,241	167	1,274	4,129	566	5,608	22,286	1,323	15,206	60,973
1994	43	282	2,214	105	903	4,324	374	3,775	23,703	867	10,546	63,984
1995	46	300	2,168	99	822	4,203	372	3,894	23,025	887	10,625	62,837
Midlands												
1981-85	38	309	991	268	2,203	6,278	453	5,357	16,858	1,230	16,317	50,953
1994	26	265	1,389	188	1,212	5,023	372	3,570	16,745	904	10,166	47,587
1995	33	258	1,352	198	1,204	5,078	315	3,264	16,066	863	9,457	46,343
Southern												
1981-85	60	423	1,362	164	1,331	3,984	540	6,801	22,844	1,259	18,237	60,938
1994	45	392	2,706	104	748	3,786	340	3,521	20,376	778	9,844	56,810
1995	58	442	3,014	88	703	3,649	337	3,502	20,281	783	9,690	56,539
London												
1981-85	6	35	266	56	413	2,489	301	4,269	25,584	521	7,588	45,274
1994	4	54	407	42	637	4,406	137	2,857	19,368	264	5,638	38,407
1995	4	41	317	25	640	4,349	102	2,962	18,945	200	5,899	37,857

A14: Distribution of accidents by road class and Highways Agency Region: 1994, 1995

percentage (row sums = 100)

	Motorways		Trunk roads		Principal roads		Other Roads	
	1994	1995	1994	1995	1994	1995	1994	1995
Northern	3.5	3.5	6.8	6.7	37.0	36.6	52.7	53.2
Midlands	2.9	2.9	10.6	11.0	35.2	34.7	51.3	51.5
Southern	4.8	5.3	6.7	6.5	35.9	35.9	52.7	52.3
London	1.1	0.8	11.5	11.5	50.4	50.0	37.0	37.6

A15: **Motor vehicles, population, area and road length (motorways and built-up and non built-up roads: by trunk and principal): by Highways Agency Region: 1995**

Thousands/ number

	Motor vehicles currently licensed (thousands)	Population[1] mid year (home) (thousands)	Area in hectares (thousands)	Road length (kilometres)					
				Motorways[2][3]	Built-up[3]		Non built-up[3]		
					Trunk	Principal	Trunk	Principal	
Northern	6,100	15,492	4,080	1,012	348	3,849	2,218	4,575
Midlands	5,910	12,232	4,507	663	217	2,276	2,635	4,960
Southern	7,036	14,017	4,298	1,011	117	3,102	1,820	5,568
London	2,684	6,967	158	62	203	1,358	123	44

1 Final 1994 population estimates.
2 Excluding slip roads.
3 As at April 1995. Road length figures taken from DOT Transport Statistics Report "Road Lengths in Great Britain 1995".

A16: **Motor traffic distribution between Highways Agency Region: by motorway and built-up and non built-up trunk and principal roads: 1993-1995 average**

Percentage[1]

	Motorways	Built-up A		Non built-up A		All major roads
		Trunk	Principal	Trunk	Principal	
Northern	30	25	33	27	26	29
Midlands	25	24	22	36	30	27
Southern	42	11	28	31	44	35
London	3	40	18	6	1	8

1 Figures have been rounded to the nearest whole number.

A17: **Motor traffic distribution between motorways, built-up and non built-up trunk and principal roads: by Highways Agency Region[1]: 1993-1995 average**

Percentage[1]

	Motorways	Built-up A		Non built-up A		All major roads
		Trunk	Principal	Trunk	Principal	
Northern	28	3	30	19	20	100
Midlands	25	3	21	28	24	100
Southern	32	1	21	19	27	100
London	10	16	57	14	2	100

1 Figures have been rounded to the nearest whole number.

ANNEX B

LOCAL HIGHWAY AUTHORITIES WITHIN EACH GOVERNMENT OFFICE REGION.

North East

Cleveland
Durham
Northumberland
Tyne and Wear

North West

Cheshire
Cumbria
Greater Manchester
Lancashire

Merseyside

Knowsley
Liverpool
St. Helens
Sefton
Wirral

Yorkshire and Humberside

Humberside
North Yorkshire
South Yorkshire
West Yorkshire

East Midlands

Derbyshire
Leicestershire
Lincolnshire
Northamptonshire
Nottinghamshire

West Midlands

Hereford and Worcester
Shropshire
Staffordshire
Warwickshire
West Midlands

South West

Avon
Cornwall
Devon
Dorset
Gloucestershire
Somerset
Wiltshire

Eastern

Bedfordshire
Cambridgeshire
Essex
Hertfordshire
Norfolk
Suffolk

London

City of London
Barking
Barnet

Brent
Bromley
Camden
Croydon
Ealing

Enfield
Greenwich
Hackney
Hammersmith
Harringey

Harrow
Havering
Hillingdon
Hounslow
Islington

Kensington and Chelsea
Kingston upon Thames
Lambeth
Lewisham
Merton

Newham
Redbridge
Richmond upon Thames
Southwark
Sutton

Tower Hamlets
Waltham Forest
Wandsworth
Westminster

South East

Berkshire
Buckinghamshire
East Sussex
Hampshire
Isle of Wight
Kent
Oxfordshire
Surrey
West Sussex

Government Office Regions

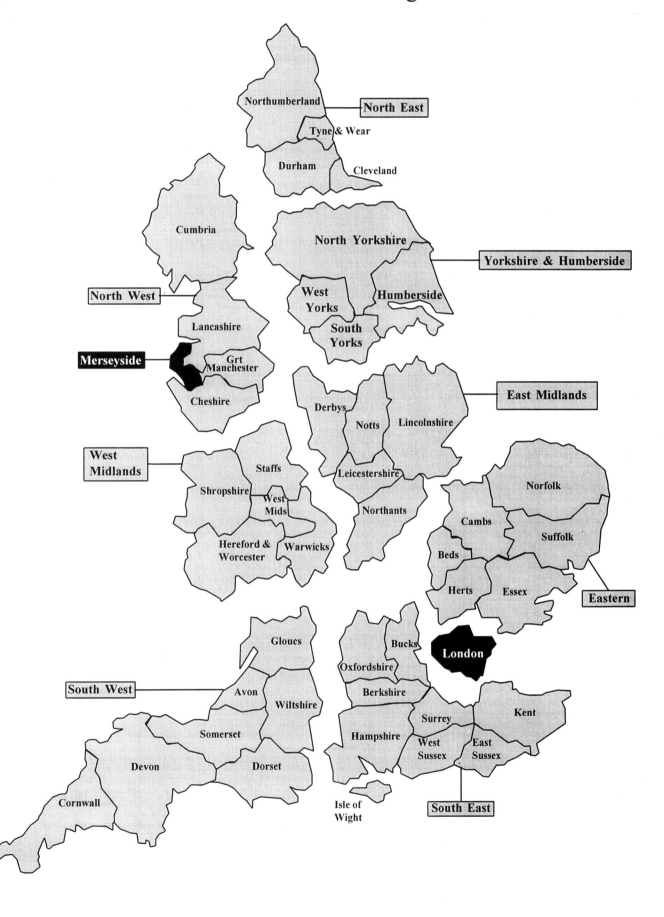

ANNEX C

LOCAL HIGHWAY AUTHORITIES WITHIN THE HIGHWAYS AGENCY NETWORK MANAGEMENT DIVISIONS

Northern

Cheshire
Cleveland
Cumbria
Derbyshire
Durham
Greater Manchester

Humberside
Lancashire
Merseyside
North Yorkshire
Northumberland

South Yorkshire
Tyne and Wear
West Yorkshire

Midland

Bedfordshire
Cambridgeshire
Gloucestershire
Hereford and Worcester

Leicestershire
Lincolnshire
Norfolk
Northamptonshire
Nottinghamshire

Oxfordshire
Shropshire
Staffordshire
Suffolk

Warwickshire
West Midlands

Southern

Avon
Berkshire
Buckinghamshire
Cornwall
Devon

Dorset
East Sussex
Essex
Hampshire
Hertfordshire

Isle of Wight
Kent
Somerset
Surrey
West Sussex

Wiltshire
London M25

London

City of London
Barking
Barnet

Brent
Bromley
Camden
Croydon
Ealing

Enfield
Greenwich
Hackney
Hammersmith
Harringey

Harrow
Havering
Hillingdon
Hounslow
Islington

Kensington and Chelsea
Kingston upon Thames
Lambeth
Lewisham
Merton

Newham
Redbridge
Richmond upon Thames
Southwark
Sutton

Tower Hamlets
Waltham Forest
Wandsworth
Westminster

HIGHWAYS AGENCY REGIONS

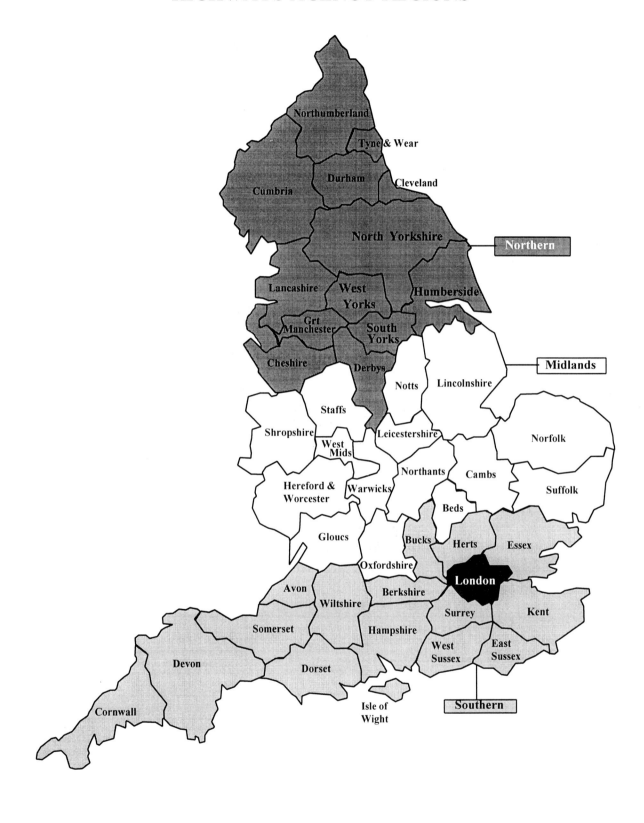

Definitions

Accident: Involves personal injury occurring on the public highway (including footways) in which a road *vehicle or pedestrian* is involved and which becomes known to the police within 30 days of its occurrence. The *vehicle* need not be moving and accidents involving stationery vehicles and pedestrians or users are included. One accident may give rise to several *casualties.* Damage-only accidents are not included in this publication.

"A" Roads: All purpose *trunk* roads and *principal* local authority roads.

Adults: Persons aged 16 years and over.

Built-up Roads: Roads with speed limits (ignoring temporary limits) of 40 mph or less. "Non built-up roads" refer to those with speed limits of over 40 mph. *Motorways* are included with non built-up roads unless otherwise stated. In tables where data for *motorways* are shown separately, the totals for built-up and non built-up roads exclude *motorway accidents*. In comparing such tables with those involving a built-up/non built-up split only, negligible error will be made by assuming that *motorway accidents* were all on non built-up roads.

Cars: Includes taxis, estate cars, invalid tricycles, three and four-wheeled cars, minibuses and motor caravans.

Casualty: A person *killed* or injured in an *accident*. Casualties are classified as either *killed, seriously injured* or *slightly injured.*

Children: Persons under 16 years of age.

Fatal accident: One in which at least one person is *killed* (but excluding confirmed suicides) and dies within 30 days of the accident.

Heavy goods vehicles (HGV): Prior to 1994 these were defined as those vehicles over 1.524 tonnes unladen weight and included vehicles with six or more tyres, some four-wheel vehicles with extra large bodies and larger rear tyres and tractor units travelling without their usual trailer. From 1 January 1994 the weight definition changed to those vehicles over 3.5 tonnes maximum permissible gross vehicle weight (gvw).

Light goods vehicles (LGV): Prior to 1994 these were defined as those vehicles not over 1.524 tonnes unladen weight. From 1 January 1994 the weight definition changed to those vehicles not over 3.5 tonnes maximum permissible gross vehicle weight. Light vans mainly include vehicles of the van type constructed on a car chassis.

Killed: Human *casualties* who sustained injuries resulting in death within 30 days of the *accident.*

KSI: *Killed* or *seriously injured.*

Licensed Vehicles: The stock of vehicles currently licensed on 31 December, when the annual census is taken at the Driver and Vehicle Licensing Agency (DVLA).

London: Where possible, data for London have been split into Inner and Outer London. Inner London comprises the City of London and the boroughs of Westminster, Camden, Islington, Hackney, Tower Hamlets, Lewisham, Southwark, Lambeth, Wandsworth, Hammersmith, Kensington and Chelsea, Newham and Haringey. Outer London is all other London boroughs, and includes Heathrow Airport. This definition conforms to that used by the Office of Population Censuses and Surveys (OPCS).

Major Roads: These are *motorways*, A(M) and *A class* roads (both *trunk* and *principal*).

Motorcyclist: Riders and passengers of two-wheeled motor vehicles.

Motorways: Motorways and A(M) roads except where otherwise noted. The motorway lengths given in Tables 15 and 17 are main line lengths and exclude associated slip roads.

Motorway Accident: *Accidents* on *motorways* include those on associated slip roads and those at junctions between *motorways* and other roads where the *accident* cannot be clearly allocated to the other road.

Other Roads: These are "B" and "C" class roads and unclassified roads, including "road class not reported".

Pedal cycle: Includes tandems, tricycles and toy cycles ridden on the carriageway. Also includes battery-assisted cycles and tricycles with a maximum speed of 15 mph.

Pedal cyclist: Riders of *pedal cycles* including any passengers.

Pedestrians: Also includes persons riding toy cycles on the footway, persons pushing bicycles or pushing or pulling other vehicles or operating pedestrian-controlled vehicles, those leading or herding animals, occupants of prams or wheelchairs, and persons who alight safely from vehicles and are subsequently injured.

Population: The population data used in calculating rates are the final mid-1994 estimates. Mid-year estimates for 1995 were not available at the time of going to publication. The estimates include residents who are temporarily outside the country, and exclude both foreign visitors and members of HM armed forces who are stationed abroad.

Principal Roads: Roads for which County Councils (Regional and Island Authorities in Scotland) are the Highway Authority. The classified *principal roads* (which include local authority *motorways*) are those of regional and urban strategic importance.

Serious Accident: One in which at least one person is *seriously injured* but no person (other than a confirmed suicide) is killed.

Serious Injury: An injury for which a person is detained in hospital as an "in-patient", or any of the following injuries whether or not the *casualty* was detained in hospital: fractures, concussion, internal injuries, crushings, severe cuts and lacerations, severe general shock requiring medical treatment, injuries causing death 30 or more days after the *accident*. An injured *casualty* is coded as seriously or *slightly injured* by the police on the basis of information available within a short time of the *accident*. This generally will not include the result of a medical examination, but may include the fact of being detained in hospital, the reasons for which may vary from area to area.

Severity: Of an *accident*, the severity of the most severely injured *casualty* (either fatal, serious or slight); of a casualty, killed, seriously injured or slightly injured.

Slight Accident: One in which at least one person is *slightly injured*, but no person is *killed* or *seriously injured*.
Slight Injury: An injury of a minor character such as a sprain, bruise or cut which are not judged to be severe, or slight shock requiring roadside attention only.

Two-wheel motor vehicles: Mopeds, motor scooters and motor cycles (including motor cycle combinations).

Trunk Roads: Roads comprising the national network of through routes for which the Secretary of State for Transport in England and the Secretaries of State for Scotland and Wales are the highway authorities. The network contains both *motorways*, which legally are special roads reserved for certain classes of traffic, and all-purpose roads which are open to all classes of traffic.

Accident Record Attendant Circumstances

1.1 Record Type
  11 New accident record
  15 Amended accident record

1.2 Police Force

1.3 Accident Ref No

1.5 Number of Vehicle Records

1.6 Number of Casualty Records

1.7 Date
  Day Month Year

1.9 Time of Day
  Hours Mins
  24 hour

1.10 Local Authority

1.11 Location
  10 digit OS Grid Reference number
  Easting
  Northing

1.12 1st Road Class
  1 Motorway
  2 A (M)
  3 A
  4 B
  5 C
  6 Unclassified

1.13 1st Road Number

1.14 Carriageway Type or Markings
  1 Roundabout - on circular highway
  2 One way street
  3 Dual carriageway - 2 lanes
  4 Dual carriageway - 3 or more lanes
  5 Single carriageway - single track road
  6 Single carriageway - 2 lanes (one in each direction)
  7 Single carriageway - 3 lanes (two way capacity)
  8 Single carriageway - 4 or more lanes (two way capacity)
  9 Unknown

1.15 Speed Limit
  mph

1.16 Junction Detail
  00 Not at or within 20 metres of junction
  01 Roundabout
  02 Mini roundabout
  03 T or staggered junction
  04 Y junction
  05 Slip road
  06 Crossroads
  07 Multiple junction
  08 Using private drive or entrance
  09 Other junction

Junction Accidents Only

1.17 Junction Control
  1 Authorised person
  2 Automatic traffic signal
  3 Stop sign
  4 Give way sign or markings
  5 Uncontrolled

1.18 2nd Road Class
  1 Motorway
  2 A (M)
  3 A
  4 B
  5 C
  6 Unclassified

1.19 2nd Road Number

1.20 Pedestrian Crossing Facilities
  00 No crossing facility within 50 metres
  01 Zebra crossing
  02 Zebra crossing controlled by school crossing patrol
  03 Zebra crossing controlled by other authorised person
  04 Pelican or puffin crossing
  05 Other light controlled crossing
  06 Other site controlled by school crossing patrol
  07 Other site controlled by other authorised person
  08 Central refuge - no other controls
  09 Footbridge or subway

1.21 Light Conditions
  1 Daylight: street lights present
  2 Daylight: no street lighting
  3 Daylight: street lighting unknown
  4 Darkness: street lights present and lit
  5 Darkness: street lights present but unlit
  6 Darkness: no street lighting
  7 Darkness: street lighting unknown

1.22 Weather
  1 Fine without high winds
  2 Raining without high winds
  3 Snowing without high winds
  4 Fine with high winds
  5 Raining with high winds
  6 Snowing with high winds
  7 Fog or mist - if hazard
  8 Other
  9 Unknown

1.23 Road Surface Condition
  1 Dry
  2 Wet / Damp
  3 Snow
  4 Frost / Ice
  5 Flood (surface water over 3cm deep)

1.24 Special Conditions at Site
  0 None
  1 Automatic traffic signal out
  2 Automatic traffic signal partially defective
  3 Permanent road signing defective or obscured
  4 Road works present
  5 Road surface defective

1.25 Carriageway Hazards
  0 None
  1 Dislodged vehicle load in carriageway
  2 Other object in carriageway
  3 Involvement with previous accident
  4 Dog in carriageway
  5 Other animal or pedestrian in carriageway

1.27 DOT Special Projects

Vehicle Record

2.1 Record Type
21 New vehicle record
25 Amended vehicle record

2.2 Police Force

2.3 Accident Ref No

2.4 Vehicle Ref No

2.5 Type of Vehicle
01 Pedal cycle
02 Moped
03 Motor scooter
04 Motor cycle
05 Combination
06 Invalid tricycle
07 Other three-
    wheeled car
08 Taxi
09 Car (four-wheeled)
10 Minibus / Motor caravan
11 Bus or coach
12 Light goods vehicle
13 Heavy goods vehicle
14 Other motor vehicle
15 Other non-motor vehicle

2.6 Towing and Articulation
0 No tow or articulation
1 Articulated vehicle
2 Double or multiple trailer
3 Caravan
4 Single trailer
5 Other tow

2.7 Manoeuvres
01 Reversing
02 Parked
03 Waiting to go ahead but held up
04 Stopping
05 Starting
06 U turn
07 Turning left
08 Waiting to turn left
09 Turning right
10 Waiting to turn right
11 Changing lane to left
12 Changing lane to right
13 Overtaking moving vehicle on its offside
14 Overtaking stationary vehicle on its offside
15 Overtaking on nearside
16 Going ahead left hand bend
17 Going ahead right hand bend
18 Going ahead other

2.8 Vehicle Movement Compass Point
From To
Parked: not at kerb 0 0
at kerb * 0
* code 1 - 8

1 N
2 NE
3 E
4 SE
5 S
6 SW
7 W
8 NW

2.9 Vehicle Location at Time of Accident
01 Leaving the main road
02 Entering the main road
03 On the main road
04 On the minor road
05 On service road
06 On lay-by or hard shoulder
07 Entering lay-by or hard shoulder
08 Leaving lay-by or hard shoulder
09 On cycleway
10 Not on carriageway

2.10 Junction Location of Vehicle at First Impact
0 Not at junction (or within 20 metres)
1 Vehicle approaching junction or parked at junction approach
2 Vehicle in middle of junction
3 Vehicle cleared junction or parked at junction exit
4 Did not impact

2.11 Skidding and Overturning
0 No skidding, jack-knifing or overturning
1 Skidded
2 Skidded and overturned
3 Jack-knifed
4 Jack-knifed and overturned
5 Overturned

2.12 Hit Object in Carriageway
00 None
01 Previous accident
02 Road works
03 Parked vehicle - lit
04 Parked vehicle - unlit
05 Bridge - roof
06 Bridge - side
07 Bollard / Refuge
08 Open door of vehicle
09 Central island of roundabout
10 Kerb
11 Other object

2.13 Vehicle Leaving Carriageway
0 Did not leave carriageway
1 Left carriageway nearside
2 Left carriageway nearside and rebounded
3 Left carriageway straight ahead at junction
4 Left carriageway offside onto central reservation
5 Left carriageway offside onto central reservation and rebounded
6 Left carriageway offside and crossed central reservation
7 Left carriageway offside
8 Left carriageway offside and rebounded

2.14 Hit Object Off Carriageway
00 None
01 Road sign / Traffic signal
02 Lamp post
03 Telegraph pole / Electricity pole
04 Tree
05 Bus stop / Bus shelter
06 Central crash barrier
07 Nearside or offside crash barrier
08 Submerged in water (completely)
09 Entered ditch
10 Other permanent object

2.16 First Point of Impact
0 Did not impact
1 Front
2 Back
3 Offside
4 Nearside

2.17 Other Vehicle Hit
Ref no of other vehicle

2.18 Part(s) Damaged
0 None
1 Front
2 Back
3 Offside
4 Nearside
5 Roof
6 Underside
7 All four sides

2.21 Sex of Driver
1 Male
2 Female
3 Not traced

2.22 Age of Driver
Estimated if necessary
Years

2.23 Breath Test
0 Not applicable
1 Positive
2 Negative
3 Not requested
4 Failed to provide
5 Driver not contacted at time

2.24 Hit and Run
0 Other
1 Hit and Run
2 Non-stop, vehicle not hit

2.25 DOT Special Projects

2.26 Vehicle Registration Mark (VRM)
VRM or one of the following codes
2 Foreign / Diplomatic
3 Military
4 Trade plates
9 Unknown

Casualty Record

3.1 Record Type
[3]

31 New casualty record
35 Amended casualty record

3.2 Police Force

3.3 Accident Ref No

3.4 Vehicle Ref No

3.5 Casualty Ref No

3.6 Casualty Class

1 Driver or rider
2 Vehicle or pillion passenger
3 Pedestrian

3.7 Sex of Casualty

1 Male
2 Female

3.8 Age of Casualty

Years

Estimated if necessary

3.9 Severity of Casualty

1 Fatal
2 Serious
3 Slight

3.10 Pedestrian Location

00 Not a pedestrian
01 In carriageway, crossing on pedestrian crossing
02 In carriageway, crossing within zig-zag lines at crossing approach
03 In carriageway, crossing within zig-zag lines at crossing exit
04 In carriageway, crossing elsewhere within 50 metres of pedestrian crossing
05 In carriageway, crossing elsewhere
06 On footway or verge
07 On refuge, central island or central reservation
08 In centre of carriageway, not on refuge, central island or central reservation
09 In carriageway, not crossing
10 Unknown or other

3.11 Pedestrian Movement

0 Not a pedestrian
1 Crossing from driver's nearside
2 Crossing from driver's nearside - masked by parked or stationary vehicle
3 Crossing from driver's offside
4 Crossing from driver's offside - masked by parked or stationary vehicle
5 In carriageway, stationary - not crossing (standing or playing)
6 In carriageway, stationary - not crossing (standing or playing), masked by parked or stationary vehicle
7 Walking along in carriageway - facing traffic
8 Walking along in carriageway - back to traffic
9 Unknown or other

3.12 Pedestrian Direction

Compass point bound

1 N
2 NE
3 E
4 SE
5 S
6 SW
7 W
8 NW
0 Standing still

3.13 School Pupil Casualty

1 School pupil on journey to or from school
0 Other

3.15 Car Passenger

0 Not a car passenger
1 Front seat car passenger
2 Rear seat car passenger

3.16 Bus or Coach Passenger

0 Not a bus or coach passenger
1 Boarding
2 Alighting
3 Standing passenger
4 Seated passenger

3.17 DOT Special Projects

Printed in the United Kingdom for HMSO
Dd 303058 C6 8/96